MY AWESOME GUIDE TO FRESHWATER FISHING

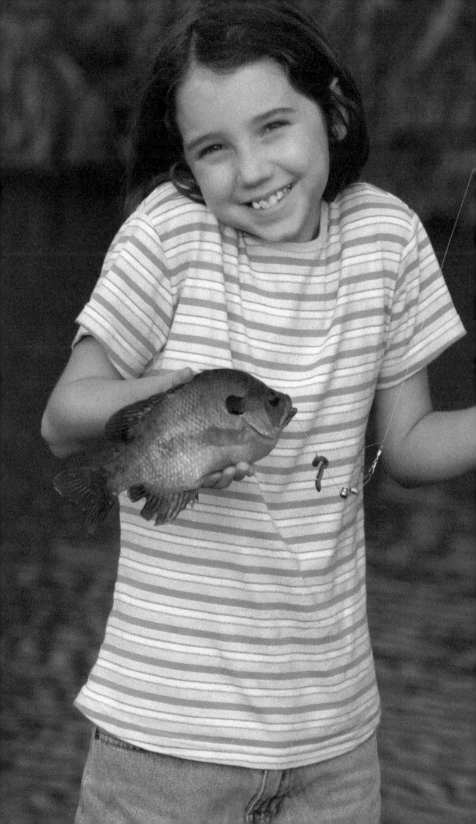

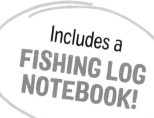

Includes a
FISHING LOG
NOTEBOOK!

My Awesome

GUIDE TO

FRESHWATER FISHING

Essential Techniques and Tools for Kids

JOHN PAXTON

Illustrations by Monika Melnychuk

ROCKRIDGE
PRESS

Series Designer: Josh Moore
Interior and Cover Designer: Patricia Fabricant
Art Producer: Sue Bischofberger
Editor: Andrea Leptinsky
Illustration © 2021 Monika Melnychuk
Cover and interior photography used under license from iStockphoto.com and shutterstock.com

Paperback ISBN: 978-1-64876-890-3
eBook ISBN: 978-1-64876-891-0
R0

For Tristan and Amber

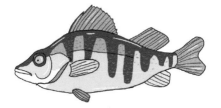

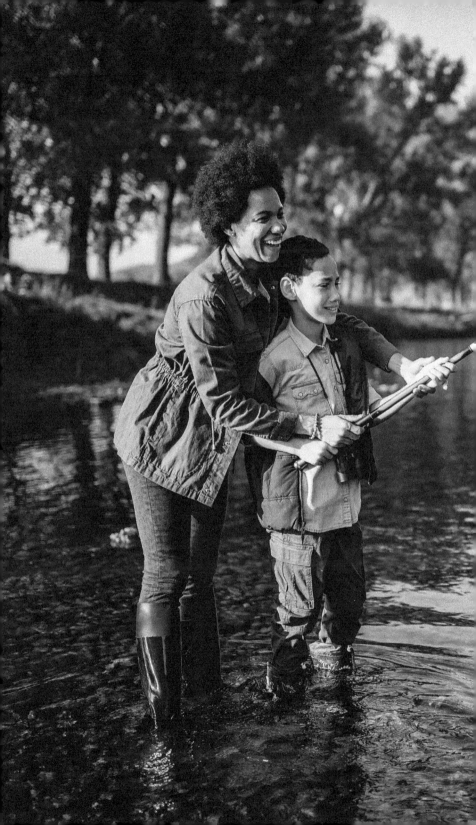

Contents

Welcome, Anglers!

Hi! My name is John Paxton, and I can't wait to help you learn how to fish. Fishing has always been a huge part of my life. There are photos of me with a giant smile on my face, looking at a fish my dad caught, when I could not have been much older than two. Some of my earliest memories are of trips to the local fish hatchery with my grandparents and fishing with my dad at a park. When I was about five, my dad bought a house on Lake Champlain with his friend. That was more than 30 years ago and I've spent most of each summer there since.

I taught my children how to fish and want to teach others, too. I created a website to help people learn about this sport. Now, I wrote this book for you. The skills I teach you will help you have many fishing adventures throughout your life that you can share with friends and family. You'll see more beautiful sunrises and sunsets than you can imagine, and breathe the crisp air only found on the water. You will become more connected with the Earth as you tune into nature and its seasons. It's going to be great!

My goal is for this book to be a handy reference that you can keep in your **tackle** box to help you catch fish most of the times you go out. I hope this book helps you make many happy memories out on the water, and that you come to love fishing as much as I do. So, why do I love fishing?

I love fishing because it is so unpredictable. I might catch 100 fish one day, while barely getting a bite the next. Anytime I cast, I never know what might **strike**. It could be a tiny bluegill, or a massive northern pike.

I love fishing because it is exciting. There's nothing quite like working a **topwater lure** near a weed edge, only to see a giant bulge in the water headed straight for it, then the huge splash of water from the strike. That thrill beats anything you can find in a video game.

Above all else, I love fishing because it is one of very few sports that *anyone* can participate in. You don't have to be rich to catch fish. It doesn't matter where you're from or who you are. You can fish standing up, sitting down, or even lying on your side, if you really feel like it. You can be young, old, or anything in between.

If you don't believe me, look up Clay Dyer. He was born without legs, hands, and most of his arms, yet he fulfilled his dream of becoming a professional **angler** and inspires everyone who meets him.

Fishing is for everyone, so let's make fishing for you.

Note to Parents

If you're a parent reading this book, go ahead and breathe a sigh of relief. In an age when every kid seems glued to a screen, yours is excited to go fishing outside. As they explore this hobby, they'll breathe fresh air, develop a love for the great outdoors, and learn a valuable life skill that can help sustain their mind and body.

There's only one catch: Fishing can be *difficult*. You know that pit in your stomach you get when your child is playing Little League baseball and they strike out? Fishing can be like that, with every cast. Managing their attitude, and your own, is even more important than finding fish. That's where you come in. When your child is just starting out, remember these three tips:

→ Try to get a fish, frog, turtle, or crayfish in the live well, or bucket, as soon as possible.

→ Fish in places that have a "Plan B," like a playground, or bring something with you, like a soccer ball, for an alternate activity.

→ Control what you can control: Bring snacks, sunscreen, a first aid kit, and a great attitude.

If you do these three things, you'll have a day full of great memories—whether you catch any fish or not.

Throughout this book, you'll see a little 🛡 indicating an important safety tip to follow. Fishing is a sport that involves many sharp objects, such as hooks and teeth. While I've done my best to write a book that is accessible to all ages, you're the best judge of what tasks your child is ready for and what items they'll need help with to prevent an accident.

Note to Kids

I hope you're as excited to read this book as I was to write it. Fishing is an incredibly fun sport that allows you to connect with nature and learn skills that are useful in life. In this book, you'll learn what makes a great fishing spot, what types of lures and baits you should use for different fish, and how to cast, hook, and land your next trophy.

Not only is fishing fun, but it's also a hobby that can open doors for you. Many colleges offer fishing scholarships. The fishing industry supports jobs in marketing, sales, journalism, and science. Even if you don't want a career in fishing, the skills you learn, such as patience, research, and perseverance, will come in handy every day.

One thing I wish I had done more as a kid was keep track of which fish I caught and where. I started doing this later in life and find it helpful to have a record to refer to. Luckily for you, there's a fishing log included at the end of this book. Record your catches there so you have something to reference when conditions are similar in the future.

SAFETY FIRST

Fishing is normally a safe sport, but it is also one that requires you to regularly handle sharp objects and unpredictable, live animals. If you aren't paying attention, things can go wrong. Make sure you pay attention to the **SAFETY TIPS** when they appear in this book. To start, here are seven quick tips to keep you safe while you are on the water.

→ Take your time. You are far more likely to be injured while rushing.

→ Always wear sunscreen, a hat, and sunglasses. You won't find much shade while fishing and you can be burned badly unless you're wearing proper sun gear. Sunglasses will also protect your eyes if your fishing buddy makes a bad cast.

→ Pinch the barbs down on hooks. This means taking pliers, holding them so they grab the hook point, and then pinching the barb until it is bent. This way, if an accident happens, it won't hurt so bad.

→ Use monofilament fishing line. Braid fishing line is stronger, but it can cut you badly if you're holding on to it and a fish starts to run.

→ Know how to hold a fish before you grab it. Some fish have very sharp teeth or spines. Think about buying a pair of fish grippers to help you bring in your fish safely.

If you're fishing from a boat, there are two very important safety tips you need to know:

→ Always wear your life jacket.

→ When the motor is on, the boat's driver should always wear the kill switch. This is a key attached to a rope that is tied to the driver's life jacket. If the driver falls out of the boat, the key will come out and the engine will turn off.

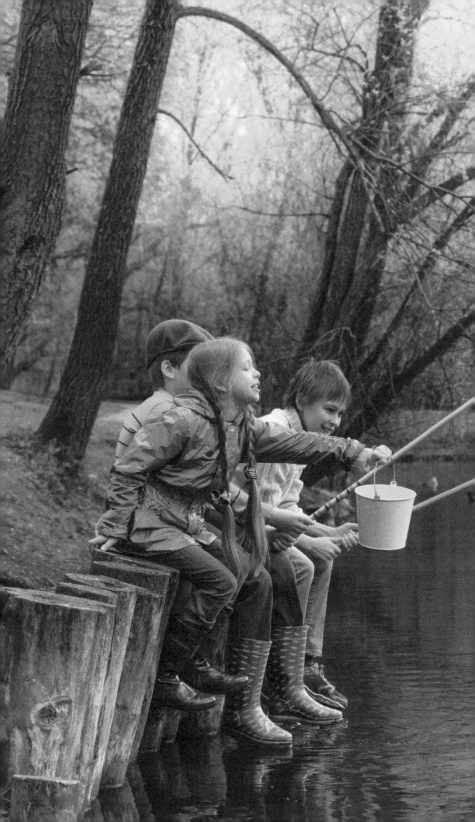

CHAPTER ONE
Tools of the Trade

I was a kid reading a book like this once, so I know the deal. You're probably tempted to jump right to chapters 2 or 3 and ignore this one, but that would be a mistake. In this chapter, you'll learn all about the different tools you'll use while fishing: rods, reels, lines, lures, and bait. We're starting here because it's important. You don't want to hook the biggest fish of your life only to find that your tackle can't hold up to it or have your knot slip. If you skip ahead, that may be exactly what happens.

ABRAHAM LINCOLN REPORTEDLY
said, "Give me six hours to cut down a tree, and I'll spend the first four sharpening the axe." Think of reading this chapter as sharpening your axe. Once you understand all the different fishing tools and how they work together, you'll have much greater success catching a fish.

What's in Your Tackle Box

Fishing is a huge business with billions of dollars in sales every year. It's no wonder that every tackle shop is packed with hundreds of fishing lures, rods, reels, gadgets, and tools. With so many options for each of these things, it can be hard to choose what to buy. It's best to keep things simple when you're starting out. If you buy these 10 items, you'll be able to handle most situations:

→ Fishing license (if required)
→ Spinning rod and reel
→ 6 lb. test monofilament fishing line
→ A few hooks small enough for sunfish to bite
→ Some bait (worms or corn where legal)
→ A few bobbers
→ Some sinkers (nuts and bolts will do in a pinch)
→ A few lures (I suggest spinnerbaits)
→ Needle-nose pliers with a line cutter
→ A tackle bag or box to hold all these things

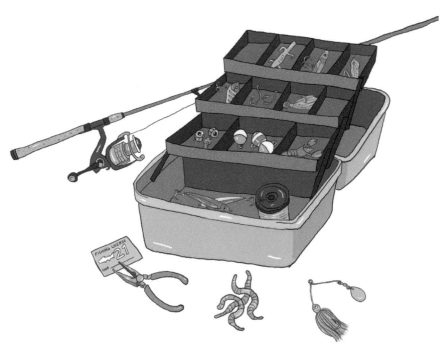

While it's fun to think about tackle, don't forget the following items. They might seem boring compared to a flashy spinnerbait, but leaving any of these at home might ruin your day. Fishing isn't much fun on an empty stomach while you're getting soaked by rain.

→ Rubber net
→ Proper sun gear (hat, sunglasses, and sunscreen)
→ Rain gear
→ Water and snacks

> **SAFETY TIP** Remember that some of the items listed are sharp. Pay attention to what you're doing, take your time, and ask an adult for help if you aren't comfortable handling any of this gear.

DO I NEED A FISHING LICENSE?

Most states allow younger children to fish for free, but depending on your age and where you live, you may need a fishing license to fish legally. Don't worry. There's no test, just a small fee. You can buy a fishing license at most tackle shops, sporting goods stores, and even your town hall. Licenses are issued by your local government, and the money is usually used to protect fish habitats. Fishing laws change now and then, so make sure to check with your state's fish and wildlife agency before you fish.

Sometimes states will have a "free fishing day" when you don't need to have a license to fish. This is a great way to figure out if this sport is for you or to introduce a friend to fishing. Check with your local government to see if any such days are planned in your state.

There is one more important thing to note about licenses. Make sure that your fishing license covers the kind of fishing you want to try. In my state, I need separate licenses for freshwater, saltwater, and river fishing. As always, check your local rules.

Poles, Rods, and Reels

You've probably heard people talk about both their fishing pole and fishing rod. Did you know that these aren't the same thing? Fishing poles can be quite simple. Basically, they're just sticks of some sort with a line tied to the top. You can make your own at home easily. I'll even show you how a little later. Fishing rods, on the other hand, are complex tools designed to be used with a fishing reel. Most anglers use fishing rods because they are useful in many situations.

RODS

Rods are made of a few parts: the handle, reel seat, blank, tip, and guides.

→ **Handle:** This is where your hand goes. Handles are made from different materials such as wood, cork, or heavy-duty foam. A wooden handle lets you "feel" a fish on the line better, but cork and foam are more comfortable and easier to use in the rain.

→ **Reel Seat:** This is where you attach the fishing reel. If you hold a rod straight out in front of you, a spinning rod's reel seat is underneath, and a casting or spincasting rod's reel seat is on the top.

→ **Blank:** The blank is the rod itself. Blanks can also be made from different materials, but most these days are either fiberglass or graphite.

→ **Tip:** This is the very tip of the blank. It is the most sensitive part of the rod and can break easily. Be careful when handling this part of the rod, and never reel a fish all the way to the tip.

→ **Guides:** Fishing rods have several loops or circles attached to them. These are the line guides, also called **eyes**. You string your line through these from the reel to the tip. The smaller the guides, the more accurate the cast.

If you've ever gone to a tackle shop, you were probably amazed at just how many fishing rods are out there. They come in all sizes and colors. If you look closely, most have a label on them with a curious phrase like "Medium-Heavy Power, Fast Action." This label has important information that will help you choose the best rod for the type of fish you want to catch and the lures you'll need to do that.

→ **Length:** This is how long the rod is. A longer rod will cast farther and give you better control over a fish, but it is harder to cast correctly.

→ **Power:** A rod's power is how strong it is. Try to match the rod's power with the type of fish you want to catch. For example, an ultralight rod makes fishing for bluegills fun, but you would have a hard time handling a northern pike with it.

→ **Action:** A rod's action is how far up the blank it bends. Actions range from slow to fast.

Faster action rods bend toward the tip. Slower action rods bend closer to the reel seat.

→ **Lure Weight:** This is the size of lure that the rod can easily cast. For example, if the label says "¼ to ½ ounce" and you try to cast a ¾-ounce spinnerbait, it will feel heavy and won't cast as accurately. Also, it might even break the rod. Likewise, if you try to cast a lure that weighs less than ¼ ounce, the rod will not bend enough to cast the lure very far.

→ **Line Weight:** This is the size of fishing line that the rod can use without danger of breaking. While it isn't fun to break your line, it's much better than snapping your rod. Keep in mind that the reel's **drag** system acts as a safety, so if that is set up properly, you can get away with a little heavier line than the rod's label suggests.

SPINNING RODS

I recommend starting with a spinning rod and reel instead of a baitcaster. They are much easier to use and work well in nearly all circumstances. While they aren't as precise as a baitcaster, with time and practice you'll get the hang of it.

Spinning rods' eyes, or line guides, are located beneath the blank and point toward the ground. These rods don't have a trigger on the handle because you are supposed to hold the actual handle instead of palming the reel as with a baitcaster.

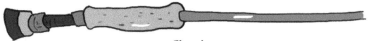

Fly rod

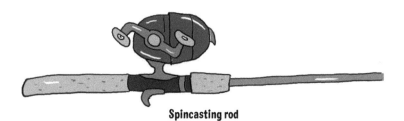

Spincasting rod

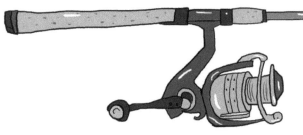

Spinning rod

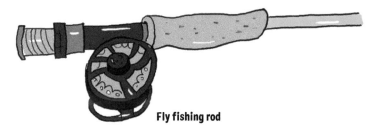

Fly fishing rod

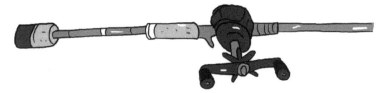

Baitcasting rod

Spinning rods are usually, but not always, lighter than baitcasters. This is because they are often used for **finesse fishing** with lighter lures and fishing line. This makes them a better choice than a baitcaster if you're going to fish with something lightweight, like a drop shot. It can be hard to find very heavy freshwater spinning rods, but there are plenty of them available for saltwater fishing. Trust me, the fish won't know the difference.

Is it okay to use a casting rod with a spinning reel and vice versa? You can certainly do this if there is no other option, but I don't recommend it. Why? Casting rods and spinning rods have eyes on opposite sides of the blanks, so using the wrong reel will make the rod flex in the opposite direction it was designed to. You could probably get away with this, but there is a chance you could damage your rod.

CASTING RODS

Casting rods are handy because they can use both baitcasting and spincasting reels. The eyes on casting rods are located on the top side. Most also have what looks like a trigger on their handle. The trigger helps you "palm" your baitcasting reel while still controlling your rod. "Palming" means holding the rod mostly by the reel, instead of by the handle. Without the trigger, it would be easy to drop your rod.

Casting rods, especially ones for freshwater, are usually heavier than spinning rods. This is because baitcasting reels are meant for bigger lures and fish. It takes a strong rod to cast larger lures and pull fish through heavy **cover**.

Casting rods come in many lengths, powers, and actions. If you can buy just one, I suggest a Medium-Heavy Power, Fast Action rod that is 6 feet 6 inches or 7 feet long. This is a good choice because you can use many common lure types with it and in many situations. Casting rods work just as well with plastic worms as they do with spinnerbaits. They can also handle crankbaits and frogs if necessary.

As I noted earlier, casting rods and baitcasting reels are not the best choice for beginners. Because they are more advanced tools than spinning reels, they can be extremely frustrating to learn to use, are difficult to cast in windy conditions, and can easily get massive, record-breaking tangles that can ruin your entire trip.

So, why do people put up with them? Well, once you get the hang of a baitcasting rod, you'll see that it gives you much more control over your casts. There are several types of casts that work best with these rods. Once you become skilled using them, you can cast out lures that gently drop into the water with nearly no splash to scare the fish. If you find that you love fishing, you should try them eventually. I'm just warning you that if they're the first rod and reel you pick up, you might decide fishing isn't for you.

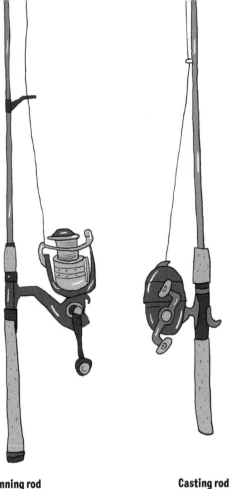

Spinning rod   **Casting rod**

REELS

There are four types of fishing reels: spincast reels, spinning reels, baitcasting reels, and fly reels. As with rods, it's important to know which reel is appropriate for the type of fishing you'll be doing.

→ **Spincast reels** are good for beginners. The fishing line is protected inside the reel, which makes tangles less likely. They are the easiest reels to cast (see chapter 3). Some spincast reels will have a difficult time with larger fish.

→ **Spinning reels** have an open spool, which means you can see the line. The spool only moves when you reel, not when you cast. They do well with lighter lines and smaller lures. Larger spinning reels can handle heavy lures. Spinning reels are a little more difficult to cast than spincast reels, but they are more versatile and usually a better option.

→ **Baitcasting reels** can cast the heaviest lures and pull the biggest fish out of cover. Unfortunately, they don't do well with light line and lures, as the line tends to tangle, making them difficult to use. Most anglers use these as their main fishing reels, but you shouldn't feel like you need to use them right away. You can perform most fishing techniques with larger spinning reels instead.

→ **Fly reels** go on fly rods and are used for catching trout and salmon in streams. I don't talk about fly fishing in this book, but it can be another fun method to try to catch fish.

Baitcasting and fly reels are very precise tools, but also difficult to use. Unless you know a skilled angler who can teach you how to use them, avoid them while you are learning. Instead, concentrate on spincast and spinning reels while you're starting out.

Once you've made a decision on which reel to use, it's time to pick out a rod. There are casting rods and spinning rods. We'll look at both.

DIY FISHING POLE

You don't have an expensive rod and reel to fish with right now? No problem; you can make your own fishing pole. All you need is a strong stick, some fishing line, and a hook.

- → Find a stick about 6 feet long that has some bend to it. Use a sapling or live tree branch instead of a dead one so it won't snap easily. You may need to sand it smooth.

- → Ask a parent to help you carve a very small notch near the tip of the stick. This will help prevent a fish from pulling the line off your pole.

- → Tie some fishing line around the notch and then tie a hook to the end of the fishing line.

- → Voilà! You just need some bait and you're ready to go fishing.

WHICH ROD IS RIGHT FOR YOU?

REEL	SPINNING	SPINCASTING	BAITCASTING	FLY
ROD	Spinning rod	Casting rod	Casting rod	Fly rod
SPOOL TYPE	Open; stationary spool beneath the rod	Enclosed; stationary spool on top of the rod	Revolving spool on top of the rod	Revolving spool beneath the rod
ACCURACY	Good accuracy	Good accuracy	High accuracy	Requires practice for accuracy
LURE SIZE/ WEIGHT	Small to medium	Small to medium	Medium to heavy	Lightweight lures like flies
EASE OF USE	Average	Easy	Difficult	Difficult
TANGLES	Knots are common	Minimal	Severe tangles are common	Unlikely
RECOMMENDATIONS	The best choice for a beginner because it has more uses than a spincaster	Probably the easiest for a beginner, but not the best choice to grow with in the sport	Not recommended for beginners	Not recommended for beginners

Fishing Line

Let's talk about what might be the most important piece of fishing equipment—the fishing line. If
it snaps, you lose your lure and your fish, so it's
important to use the right type. One end of the

fishing line is tied to your reel, and the other is tied to your lure or hook.

Lines come in different strengths, called "pound tests." A pound test is the amount of weight that will break the line. The stronger the pound test, the thicker the line. Although a thick line is useful if you're fishing for large fish, it is also easier for fish to see and avoid. So, which kind of line should you use? Let's look at the three types: braided, fluorocarbon, and monofilament.

Braided fishing line is stronger for its size than other types of line and is not very stretchy. Braid is also easy for fish to see. If you plan on fishing with braid, make sure you bring along a good pair of scissors. It can be hard to cut with a regular line cutter or pliers.

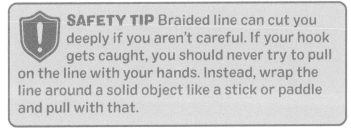

SAFETY TIP Braided line can cut you deeply if you aren't careful. If your hook gets caught, you should never try to pull on the line with your hands. Instead, wrap the line around a solid object like a stick or paddle and pull with that.

Fluorocarbon line is almost invisible underwater, and it has high abrasion resistance. This means it is hard to damage. Fluorocarbon is very stiff, which makes it hard to tie and manage. Because this line sinks, it isn't a good choice for topwater lures. Fluorocarbon line can also be expensive. I don't recommend it for beginners.

Monofilament line is the best line to use when you're starting out. It is fairly strong and comes in colors that are hard for fish to see, such as low-viz green. It is not as stiff as fluorocarbon, which makes it easier to use.

If you can buy only one spool of line to start, I recommend 6 lb. test monofilament. It is a good choice that will allow you to catch most species of fish. While 6 lb. test may seem light, if you set your reel's drag correctly, you will be able to catch heavier fish. By itself, 6 lb. test is fine for all **panfish** and most bass and pickerel that you may catch.

LEADERS

A leader is a length of material, usually metal or fluorocarbon, tied to the end of your fishing line. The lure is tied to the end of the leader. Leaders come in handy when you are trying to catch a fish with sharp teeth (a good time for a metal leader), or when you're fishing in clear water and don't want fish to see your line (a fluorocarbon leader will help with this).

You should always try to use the smallest leader possible. Large, heavy leaders can hurt a lure's action and make it more difficult to catch fish. On the other hand, hooking a fish without a leader won't do you much good if the fish can bite through the line and get away.

Fishing line is tied directly onto the reel's spool. Make sure you load the line correctly. This will reduce tangles and make it easier to cast.

Follow these steps to spool line onto a spinning reel:

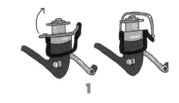

1. Make sure that the **bail** of your reel is open.

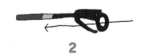

2. Run the fishing line through your line guides from the tip of the rod to the reel.

3. Tie the line to the reel and pull it tightly. I suggest an arbor knot for this.

4. Soak the spool in water to prep the fishing line.

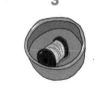

5. Reel in the line slowly while pinching it a few inches above the reel with your free hand. This will keep the line tight. A loose line won't spool well.

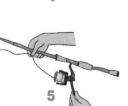

6. Don't reel in more line than the reel needs, or it will be hard to cast. A good rule of thumb is to leave about a ⅛-inch gap as shown.

Fishing Rigs

A fishing **rig** is whatever you are using on the end of your fishing line to try to catch a fish. It can be as simple as a single baited hook, or it can include a variety of hooks, lures, sinkers, or bobbers. Fishing rigs can be as complicated as you want them to be. Some anglers even use kites.

In this section, I'll discuss some of the more common items in a fishing rig. Then I'll teach you how to use my favorite rig of all: the drop shot.

HOOKS

The hook is the business end of any rig; its job is to snag the fish so you can reel it in. Hooks seem to come in as many shapes and sizes as snowflakes, so it can be hard to decide which one to use. I recommend keeping it simple. Find a hook that looks like a J to start. Try to use smaller hooks when possible. Larger ones are easier for fish to see, and harder for them to fit in their mouths.

Something that might surprise you is that larger hooks are safer than smaller ones. This is because it takes much more force to make a thicker hook pierce skin than a thin one.

> **SAFETY TIP** Hooks are very sharp and can easily poke through clothes or skin, especially if you make a sudden movement. Always approach hooks slowly and carefully. If you're uncomfortable handling them, ask an adult for help.

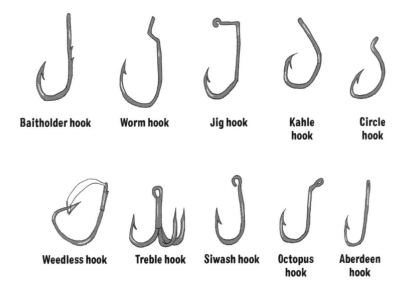

Baitholder hook   **Worm hook**   **Jig hook**   **Kahle hook**   **Circle hook**

Weedless hook   **Treble hook**   **Siwash hook**   **Octopus hook**   **Aberdeen hook**

SINKERS AND BOBBERS

Sinkers and bobbers are useful in fishing rigs because they help you put your bait at the fish's level. A sinker is a weight that you tie to your rig. If the fish are down deep, the sinker will help your bait sink quickly to where the fish can see it. A bobber does the opposite. It floats and keeps your bait higher in the water. The bobber also tells you when a fish bites. The bobber will go underwater when a fish grabs the line.

You can fine-tune your rig by adjusting how far away your bait is from a sinker or a bobber. This lets you put your lure or bait exactly where you want it.

You can certainly spend a lot of money on expensive store-bought sinkers and bobbers, but you can also make your own with what you have around the house. A nut or bolt makes a fine sinker. A small balloon makes a decent bobber; just be careful not to lose it.

KNOTS TO KNOW

Knowing how to tie knots is an important skill for any angler. There are many fishing knots, but you really only need to know five: the improved clinch knot, the Palomar knot, the uni knot, the double uni knot, and the arbor knot. I suggest practicing these with some string or shoelaces before you go fishing so that you'll be able to tie them quickly when you need to.

THE IMPROVED CLINCH KNOT

The improved clinch knot is strong and simple. It is the first knot that many anglers learn.

1. Thread the **tag end** of your fishing line through the eye of the hook.

2. Wrap the tag end around the **standing line** five or six times, leaving a large loop near the eye.

3. Push the tag end through the loop near the eye.

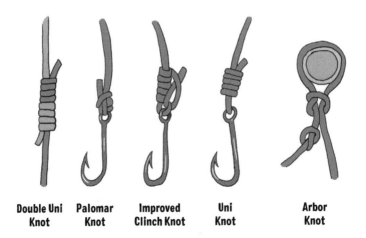

Double Uni Knot	Palomar Knot	Improved Clinch Knot	Uni Knot	Arbor Knot

4. Bring the tag end under the second large loop that you just created.

5. Tighten the knot by pulling on both ends of the line. You might need to moisten the line to do this.

THE PALOMAR KNOT

There's an old joke among bass anglers that the only knot they know is the Palomar knot because it's the only knot they need. While you can tie on any lure with a Palomar knot, it is especially useful for creating a drop shot rig (see "A Few Simple Rigs," page 24).

1. Thread the tag end of your line through the eye of the hook. Then pass it back through the eye to create a loop on one side of the eye, and a double line on the other.

2. Take the loop and tie a loose overhand knot around the double line. For this, take the loop end and place it under the double line to create a circle shape. Bring the loop end over the double line and through the circle to complete the knot.

3. Carefully, pass your hook through the loop.

4. Hold the hook firmly in one hand and pull the doubled standing line to tighten.

THE UNI KNOT

This is my favorite knot. It is quick and easy to tie.

1. Thread the tag end of the line through the eye of the hook. Then make a loop that goes over the tag and standing line.

2. Wrap the tag line through this loop and around the standing line six or seven times.

3. Pull the tag line tight to create a knot.

4. Carefully hold the hook in one hand and pull on the standing line until the knot is snug against the hook.

THE DOUBLE UNI KNOT

A double uni knot is useful for joining two types of line together, such as when you want to use a leader. I often use it when fishing with braid for this reason.

1. Lay the two different lines next to each other so the tag ends are facing opposite directions.

2. Use the tag end of one line to make a loop that goes over both lines.

3. Wrap the tag end through this loop and around the other line three or four times.

4. Pull the tag end tight.

5. Repeat steps 2 through 4 with the other line.

6. Pull the two standing lines away from each other until the two knots are tight.

THE ARBOR KNOT

This knot is used to tie your fishing line to your reel's spool. While you could use any knot for this, the arbor is strong and easy to tie.

1. Wrap your line around the spool. Then tie an overhand knot around the standing line with the tag end.

2. Tie a second overhand knot near the tag end.

3. Pull on the tag line toward the reel to tighten the two knots.

4. Tug on the main line until the two knots are snug against the spool.

A FEW SIMPLE RIGS

Now that we've discussed gear and knots, let's talk about how to put them together into two simple rigs.

The Drop Shot

If you have time to learn only one rig, I suggest the drop shot. It will catch all types of fish and is extremely easy to tie. All you have to do is tie an oversized Palomar knot, leaving a long tag end—12 inches works well. Then, tie a sinker to the tag end. This creates a rig that keeps your hook about a foot above the sinker. It will sink down to the fish, yet stay off the bottom, which helps fish see the rig. Get ready to hold on!

To fish with this rig, cast it, then simply give your line tip a few short taps while you slowly reel in the rig. Pause every so often and wait for a bite. If it is a windy day or you are fishing in a current, leave the rig in one place and wait for fish to come investigate. The waves or current do a great job of moving the lure ever so slightly, which drives fish crazy.

Sometimes the weight on a drop shot can scare the fish a little bit, and you won't get as many bites. Try removing the sinker for a few casts and see if you catch more fish. The bait will slowly drop through the water and attract the fishes' attention.

You can use a drop shot with almost any plastic lure, but my favorites are small minnow-shaped lures, and live bait such as worms. A drop shot will work well anywhere that there isn't heavy cover. If you fish around rocks, be prepared to snag the bottom often and need to retie the rig.

The Wacky Rig

True to its name, this rig looks like it was made by someone who was just joking around or not even trying, but bass love it. Just take a plastic worm, the straighter the better, and hook it directly in the center. Then, toss it into the water and let it slowly sink. If it hits bottom, lift your rod tip up and then slowly drop it again so the worm can fall a second time.

There's something about both ends of the worm flopping about that makes bass really want to bite. This rig is particularly useful in the spring during the **spawn**. If you cast a wacky rig near one of their beds, the bass find it nearly irresistible.

Bait and Lures

Now that you know all about the gear you need for fishing, how do you attract fish to bite your hook? With bait and lures. Fishing bait and lures are not the same thing. Bait is something that the fish can eat, while a lure is an artificial object meant to trick fish into thinking it is something good to eat. For example, a live worm is bait, but a plastic worm is a lure.

BAIT

Anything a fish could eat can be used as bait, whether that is corn, bread, worms, crickets, or minnows. Bait is great for catching fish because it is natural. It smells like food, looks like food, and feels like food because it *is* food. Live bait is also, well, alive. It will wriggle around all on its own, attracting fish. Because of all these things, bait is often more successful than lures.

Bait definitely has some downsides. For one, it can be very messy and smelly. Worms get dirt everywhere and minnow scales are hard to clean off equipment and your hands. Live bait is usually killed when a fish bites it. Sometimes the fish is also injured or even killed by swallowing the bait with the hook. If you find this upsetting, you should consider using lures instead.

What about bait that isn't alive? Corn is a popular choice for anglers. So is bread. Make sure to check with your local government before using these types of bait. Some states consider these to be litter and don't allow people to fish with them.

Have you ever heard someone talk about stink bait? Catfish and bullhead love smelly, gross, disgusting bait like rotting fish or chicken liver. Sometimes you don't even need to use the fish or liver. You can just soak a small sponge in the juices and put it on the hook. Be patient if you use stink bait because it may take a little while for fish to smell it and come eat it.

One way to draw fish to your location is to **chum** the water with extra bait. With luck, you could create a feeding frenzy. Be careful to check your local fishing laws to make sure it's legal. Like corn or bread, some states consider chum to be litter.

LURES

Lures are basically artificial bait. They are usually made of plastic, metal, or wood, and come in all different shapes, colors, and sizes. Unlike bait, lures usually need an angler's help to make them move. Depending on the lure, you can do this by reeling it in, or even by twitching your rod tip back and forth. Let's learn about some common lures.

SOFT PLASTICS

Lures made of soft plastic are designed to look like worms, bugs, little fish, or other creatures. While they won't wriggle on their own like the real thing, you can make them squirm by slowly twitching your rod tip. Some even come with different scents or flavors baked into them to help attract fish and keep their attention.

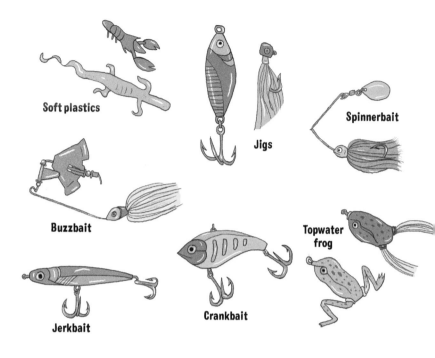

Soft plastics

Jigs

Spinnerbait

Buzzbait

Topwater frog

Jerkbait

Crankbait

Soft plastics work best when the water is a little warmer, or more than 60 degrees Fahrenheit. They are a good choice for larger fish without sharp teeth, such as largemouth and smallmouth bass. Although there are probably a million types of soft plastics to choose from, I recommend that you start with ones that look like worms. Worms are meant to crawl past fish so they can't help but bite. Precise casting will help you have success with these lures.

JIGS

The simplest jig is a hook with a weighted head. Some have plastic skirts, and others are bare hooks that you use with your favorite soft plastic lure.

To fish with a jig, you cast it out, and then slowly reel it in while raising your rod tip up and then lowering it back down. This makes the jig "pop" as it travels through the water.

Jigs can catch enormous fish, but they can be difficult for beginners to use. They're challenging because it can take a while to learn how they feel underwater. They also tend to be a big fish lure, which means you won't get as many bites from smaller fish.

Jigs are a good choice in cold water when fish aren't willing to chase lures. They're also a great choice during early spring if you know a spot where bass are spawning.

SPINNERBAITS

These lures are great for beginners. They are easy to throw and bring back, they don't get snarled often, and they catch giant fish. Spinnerbaits are basically jigs with a few flashy blades attached to a bent wire frame. The shiny blades vibrate and sparkle in the water, attracting the fish. To use a spinnerbait, simply cast it out as far as you can and then reel it back in. Every now and then, give it a little pop with your rod tip to try to make a fish grab it.

These lures come in many colors, but I only keep three in my tackle box: black, white, and yellow. Black spinnerbaits are good for cloudy days when they stand out more in the water. White spinner-baits work well in clear water, and yellow is best in murky water. Spinnerbaits work best when the water is warm: 60 degrees Fahrenheit or warmer. They're great for casting along the edge of a weed line, or for running past a sunken tree or brush.

You'll notice that spinnerbaits have differently shaped blades on them. Willow blades are long and narrow and look like little minnows. They flash a lot when they are pulled through the water and are best to use in clear water or during the day. Colorado blades look like circles. They don't flash as much but make vibrations in the water. Use them in murky water or at night.

BUZZBAITS

These lures are a lot like spinnerbaits, but instead of having thin blades that flash in the water, a buzzbait has a blade that acts like a propeller. The blade creates lift, which helps keep the lure on top of the water. They are very loud and obnoxious lures designed to annoy fish and make them attack. When one finally does, the strike creates a huge explosion of water that is exciting to see.

Buzzbaits work best when there is not much light, such as in the morning, the early evening, or even at night. I find that they work very well in the spring and especially in the fall. Throw them near cover and start reeling in as soon as they hit the water so they don't snag. Then, hold on!

One cool thing about buzzbaits is that they are even more effective when they start to squeak with age. The noisier, the better. Some people even leave them out in the rain or hang them in the wind to wear them down quicker.

These fat lures, sometimes called "plugs," are designed to look like little fish or crayfish. They usually have two sharp **treble hooks** attached. To use a crankbait, cast it out and then reel it back in until a fish strikes. Just be careful with these. The hooks are very thin and very sharp and can snag skin or clothes easily.

Like spinnerbaits, crankbaits are great for fishing a large area of water quickly. They are one of the best lures to cast from a boat. If you are fishing from shore, however, these lures may not be the best choice. It's tough to find shoreline fishing spots that aren't choked with weeds. Crankbaits get caught on weeds easily, which is frustrating.

Different crankbaits can be used in different water depths. Most have a clear plastic "bill"—like on a duck—stuck to the front of them. The larger the bill, the deeper the crankbait will go. This allows it to get down to where the fish are. These lures are great to use in the summertime when the fish hang out in deeper water.

JERKBAITS

A jerkbait is basically a long, skinny crankbait that is designed to look like a minnow or small fish. Its name comes from the method you should use to fish with it. After you cast it out, reel it in slowly, while jerking it through the water by twitching your rod tip. When using jerkbait, try out different patterns of twitches until you find one that works.

For example, you might try *jerk, jerk, pause; jerk, jerk, pause*. Try your best to mimic an injured fish while using this lure.

Jerkbaits are great lures to use in cold water where fish are a little slower. This is because you can let a jerkbait sit as long as you need to for a fish to see it, size it up, and decide to eat it. Often, a little twitch at just the right moment will make the fish bite. Jerkbaits also work fine when the water heats up. Be careful, though. Like crankbaits, these lures will snag summer weeds easily.

FROGS

Frogs are just what they sound like: plastic, frog-shaped lures that float on top of the water. They are great for fishing around plants and other cover because they won't snag. Frogs are perfect to use in midsummer when lakes and ponds are often full of vegetation.

I don't recommend these lures to beginners. While fishing with frogs is exciting because fish often strike them ferociously, it can be difficult to actually hook a fish and successfully reel it in with one. You will need to use a heavy rod with braided fishing line to give yourself the best chance. Sometimes even the pros miss more fish than they catch while fishing with frogs.

If you want to enjoy topwater fishing, you're much better off using a floating **plug** with treble hooks. While they may get snagged in the weeds, you'll have a much better chance of catching the fish that strike.

BACKYARD BAIT

Don't worry if you can't get to a tackle shop. You can find plenty of bait in your own backyard. Worms, crickets, and grasshoppers are all easy to find and make great bait.

The easiest time to find worms is at night, which is why they are sometimes called night crawlers. You'll want to search grassy areas that have been around for a while. Your school's soccer field might be a great spot to find them, but only if your school doesn't treat the grass with chemicals. Walk slowly so you don't scare them with your footsteps.

You can also find worms after it rains. They're easy to spot on pavement but can be hard to pick up. Try using a spatula, if you can.

Crickets are also easy to find. They like to hang out near woodpiles and decaying leaves. Crickets are also attracted to bread crumbs. Some folks create little traps for them with soda bottles. It's easy to do: Carefully cut off the top third of a plastic bottle and put some old nylon stocking in the bottom. Sprinkle some bread crumbs and sugar on the nylon, then firmly insert the neck piece of the bottle into the bottom piece. Lay the trap on its side near a woodpile. In a day or two, you'll have your bait.

Some Final Thoughts on Gear

I've spent a lot of time talking about all different kinds of gear, but don't worry if you don't have all the equipment that we discussed. You can still have fun and catch fish without all the fancy gadgets. There are plenty of people who catch fish with nothing but their bare hands. The knowledge you have in your brain and the willpower you have in your heart are way more important than what lures you have in your tackle box. Don't ever be discouraged by what you don't have; make the best of what you do have.

While you're starting out, keep things simple. Buy one or two rods that you're comfortable using. Pick a few lures and practice with them until you know them well. Don't feel as though you need to constantly switch tackle. If you're using the right kind of lure for the conditions, the fish will come.

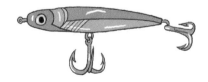

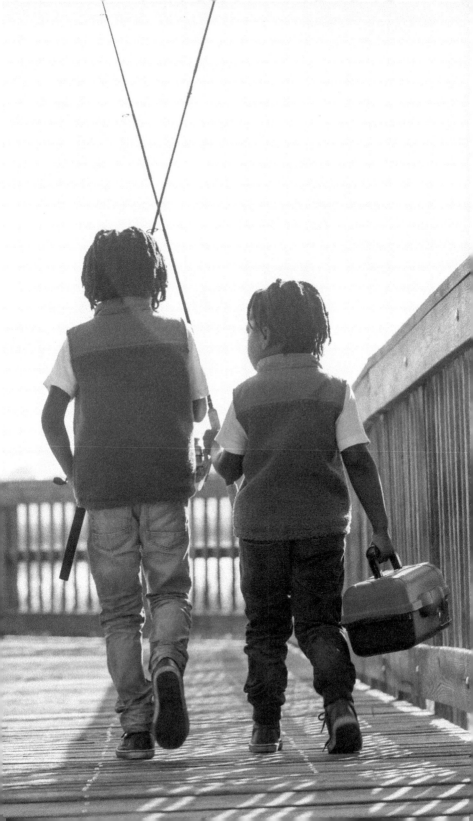

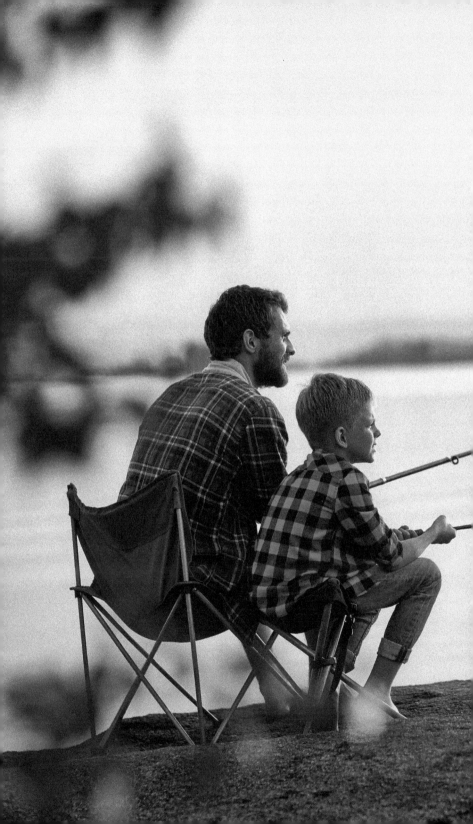

CHAPTER TWO

Where Are the Fish?

Now that you know all about fishing tools, it's time to find some fish. Where and how can you find them? Read on to find out. This chapter will focus on freshwater fishing spots. I will help you analyze your favorite pond, lake, river, or stream so you can focus on areas where fish are likely to be hanging out. This will save you time and make your fishing adventures more exciting.

YOU PROBABLY HAVE A FEW PONDS,
lakes, or rivers near you that you're thinking
of visiting. If you don't have a place in mind,
there are several organizations that can
help you find places to fish. Check out
TakeMeFishing.org, for example. Also, the
Resources section at the end of this book
provides websites that will help you find
places to fish near you.

Ponds

Most of us probably have a pond or two somewhere
near our homes. They are small bodies of water,
either man-made or natural, that are smaller
than lakes and are usually shallow. Don't let their
relatively small size make you think that only
small fish live there. Many state record—breaking
fish have come from small ponds over the years.
Even so, ponds often have large numbers of panfish, which makes them really fun to fish.

Ponds are great places to learn to fish because
you can often cover a large amount of water
simply by walking around. You don't usually need a
boat to really explore them. Even if you did, a
rubber raft would probably work well.

When you first arrive at a pond to fish, it's
helpful to walk around a little and look at the
surroundings. What are the shores like? Are they
sandy? Rocky? Woodsy? Usually, the shoreline will
give you good hints of what is beneath the

FISHING SEASONS

A fishing season is a certain time of year when people are allowed to fish. The seasons are determined by each state's government. The seasons are set up to protect the fish while they are spawning. The parent fish need to be near their young to defend them from predators. For example, in much of the northern United States, you aren't allowed to take largemouth bass until early summer, after their spawn in the spring.

Some states have created extra rules based on the different types of bodies of water. For example, in Texas, you are only allowed to take fish *over* a certain size in some lakes, but *under* a certain size in others. It can get confusing in a hurry. That's why it's important that you understand what the local rules are, so you don't get in trouble. Your state's fish and wildlife agency publishes these laws and will be happy to help you understand them.

surface. Think about the last time you were at the beach. I bet the shore was pretty sandy. It was probably sandy a good way into the water as well. Ponds work the same way. If you see lots of rocks on the shoreline, chances are there will be many underwater, too, providing great places for fish to hide.

You should also think about the time of year you'll be fishing when figuring out where to fish. In the spring, many bass and panfish stick to the warmer shallows with sandy bottoms so they can spawn. In the summer, you might need to focus on deeper, cooler water to find most fish.

Look for a stream or creek that connects to the pond. The area where the two meet, called the "mouth," can be a fantastic fishing spot. Some of the biggest fish I've caught in my life came from areas like this. These spots are particularly great in the fall. Sometimes smaller baitfish try to go up the creek at that time of year, and larger fish follow them.

One good thing to remember is that in the United States, the northwest corner of any bay or pond will warm up first in the spring. This is because it has more exposure to the sun. As mentioned in chapter 1, some lures are better when water temperatures are higher. Sometimes fast-moving lures that aren't working well on the southern end of a pond will catch tons of fish in the northwest corner.

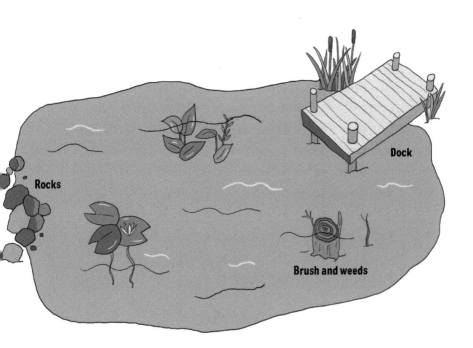

Rocks

Dock

Brush and weeds

I have one more important tip for pond fishing: Don't be afraid to go off the beaten path. Most ponds where people often fish will have certain spots that anglers like to fish from. However, those are also the places the fish might have learned to avoid. I've had great luck hiking through bushes on the bank to find a spot that not everyone fishes from. Sometimes a little effort pays off in a big way.

Lakes and Reservoirs

North America is full to the brim with natural lakes and artificial reservoirs. Many are fantastic places to catch a nice variety of fish species. You'll read about some in chapter 4. Lakes and reservoirs can be tricky to fish from shore, since there are usually only a few spots on public land. These are places where a boat makes a big difference. If you don't have a boat, don't worry. Many lakes and reservoirs have enough areas on shore to have a fun fishing trip if you know where to go.

Lakes and reservoirs are BIG, and that is what makes them challenging to fish. Not every area is going to always have tons of fish, so it is important to be thoughtful and do some research before you start fishing. The good news is that there is plenty of information on the Internet. Try simply

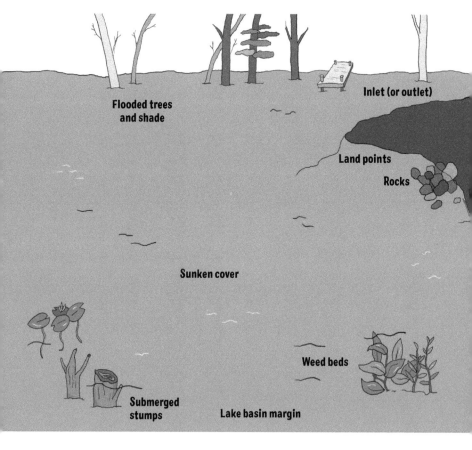

Flooded trees
and shade

Inlet (or outlet)

Land points

Rocks

Sunken cover

Weed beds

Submerged
stumps

Lake basin margin

searching for "[Lake Name] fishing reports." You should see some websites where anglers have reported on their fishing trips to that lake. Be sure to ask an adult for permission to visit these sites.

Other helpful fishing resources are navigational charts. You can probably find some online or in your local tackle shop. These charts show how deep the lake is at different points, so boats don't get stuck in shallow water. Take a look at one sometime. It can give you hints of what is hidden underwater. For example, a navigational chart will help you find underwater humps or other formations that may hold fish.

The hints I gave you for ponds are also helpful here. The northwest corner of bays, lakes, or reservoirs is going to warm the fastest, so that's a good place to start early in the year. Remember to also look for creeks or streams and focus your efforts near the mouth to increase your chances of catching a fish.

Once you find an area where lots of fish are biting, take note of what that area looks like. If there are other areas of the lake that look similar, you might try fishing them next. The log at the end of this book is a great place to write down what you see. Is there cover in the area? Is there wind? Which way is it blowing? These are all good things to remember for next time.

As I mentioned earlier, a boat is extremely helpful on a lake. But, unlike in ponds, not just any boat will always work on a lake. While a rowboat

FISHING IS FOR EVERYONE

At the very beginning of this book, I mentioned that fishing is something anyone can do—and I meant it. Modern technology and state laws help give everyone the chance to enjoy this sport.

Maybe you use a wheelchair. Many lakes and rivers have wheelchair-accessible docks, piers, and fishing spots. Your local fish and wildlife agency may have a map that shows these locations. If not, contact a local fishing club. Most local anglers also know of a few spots that would work for you. I am confident they'd be happy to share that information with a curious, well-mannered kid.

Don't forget that there are also groups that focus on helping differently abled people enjoy fishing. One such group is called Fishing Has No Boundaries. They sponsor events that help everyone get out on the water. They are listed in the Resources section at the end of this book so you can find a local chapter near your home.

or canoe is okay in the shallows of a quiet lake, many places allow large motorboats and things like jet-powered craft that can make small boats tippy. Never use a boat in a lake without an adult. If you do go fishing on a boat, a motorboat will be safer and more comfortable than a canoe or rowboat. And always wear a life jacket.

Rivers and Streams

Maybe your main places to fish are rivers and streams. In much of the country, anglers who fish in rivers are looking for trout or salmon. But if you are looking for bass, walleye, catfish, or northern pike, there are plenty of rivers that are home to those as well.

Rivers and streams can be great places to fish, but you do need to know a few things to be suc- cessful at it. You don't fish in these areas the same way you do in a lake. First, you should learn about how current affects fishing. Current is simply moving water. It can be extremely fast or very slow. Its speed usually depends on how steep the landscape of the river is. The steeper the land- scape, the faster the current. The flatter the landscape, the slower the current.

Different species of fish treat currents differ- ently. For example, smallmouth bass are often found in rivers with a fast current, while large- mouth bass prefer places where the water is much calmer. Regardless of the species, fish do their

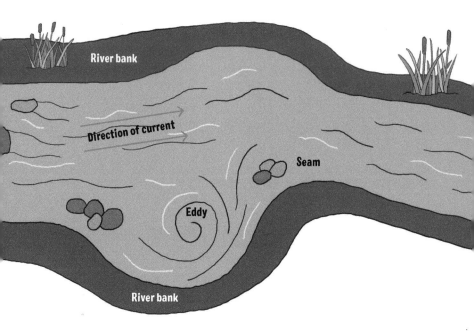

best to stay outside the current as much as they can, for example, by hiding behind a boulder. This is because it takes a lot of effort to swim in current, and effort wastes energy. Fish in the wild can't afford to waste their energy very often if they want to survive.

The fact that fish try to find places to avoid currents can help you find them in fast-moving water. Look for calm areas in the current caused by an object or change in the landscape. For example, perhaps there is a large boulder poking out of the water. While the current will move fast on either side of the boulder, there won't be any current directly behind it. That is a great place for a fish to rest and wait for some prey to be swept by. You can look for the same signs around trees that have fallen into the water or bridge pilings. Often, fish will be lurking behind these.

Very few animals are going to swim upstream, like salmon, to go after prey. Most try to preserve their energy. For this reason, you should cast upstream and guide your bait back downstream so it looks like the fish's natural prey. Try to cast in such a way that the lure will be carried past some cover or you can reel past it. Often, fish hiding behind the cover will rush out and bite the bait quickly without inspecting it because they're afraid they'll miss their chance if they don't.

Does your favorite fishing river or stream have lots of curves or bends? Then it's good for you to know that the outside bend is going to be much deeper than the inside bend. Fish tend to stay in the deeper areas, so you'll find more of them along the outside bend, or where the outside bend starts to turn into an inside bend.

Other areas that are great for fishing are pools. These are parts of a river that are deeper than their surroundings. They're caused by heavy current cutting into the riverbank. Many online forums and local publications will have good advice on where to find these near you.

Some rivers flood in the spring as melting snow mixes with seasonal rains. In some rivers, the flooded areas are great fishing spots because the water is often calmer and the shoreline's trees and bushes make fantastic cover. Unfortunately, in other rivers, floods cause stronger currents, making finding fish more difficult.

Boats are usually only allowed in large, relatively calm rivers. So, many of the rivers and streams you'll fish will require you to do it on foot. This isn't so bad because many are narrow enough that you can basically cast where you'd like. Some anglers, especially people fishing for trout, bring along a pair of waders so they can reach more spots. Waders are waterproof pants that allow you to walk into the river without getting wet. If you want to try these, always make sure you fish with an adult. Please also wear a life jacket, just in case.

SAFETY TIP Rivers can be dangerous places to fish for a few reasons. First, their currents could sweep you away if you aren't careful. Even if you could stay afloat, the current may push you into a rock or tree branch, injuring you. Current tends to get faster in areas where a river narrows, such as near bridge pilings. Second, some folks who fish rivers use something called **trotlines** dangling from trees. The hooks from these trotlines can snag unwary anglers.

Cover vs. Structure

Have you ever watched a nature program with lions and gazelles running around the African savanna? If so, have you noticed how the lions use bushes or tall grass to hide behind as they sneak up on their prey before pouncing? Fish do the same thing with underwater objects. Even though the surface of the lake or river looks flat, there's a whole underwater world filled with boulders, vegetation, and sunken objects for fish to hide near while they wait for prey. These objects are called cover.

Structure is different. The next time you take a walk, look around your neighborhood. See all the hills, valleys, ditches, and bumps? They are all examples of structure, and they also occur underwater. Structure often has cover on it. For example, an underwater hill or hump (the structure) may have some rock piles on it (the cover). Fish tend to use structure almost like a map. It helps them find their way around the lake. If you can find an interesting structure that has good cover, you will usually find fish.

Let's take some time to go over some of the covers and structures that you might find in your favorite fishing spots.

COVER

Weed beds: There are many species of weeds and aquatic plants that you might find in your local fishing hole. You might see weeds like bullrushes that stand straight up like hair coming out of the water, lily pads, and even slimy algae that look like ooze. Some plants only grow in very shallow water whereas others grow in much deeper water. Some species grow right to the water's surface and beyond, while others always stay a few feet below water.

The one thing most plant species have in common is that fish love to hide in them. Sometimes you can catch a lot of fish by running a spinnerbait down the edge of a weed line or even on top of weeds that aren't quite reaching the surface.

Rocks: Rocks and boulders tend to hold many fish, but they also are great for snagging lines and lures. Many shorelines have riprap on them, which is rock placed to prevent erosion. If you see riprap on a shoreline, chances are it extends into the water a bit. You'll find that many fish hang out in these areas, especially if the rocks are along points, which are a type of structure (see page 52).

Wood: When trees fall into water, they create the perfect habitat for fish since the cover is great for both predator and prey. Just be careful when fishing near these because if you don't get the fish away from the tree branches quickly, they can tangle your line and get away from you.

In addition to fallen trees, some man-made reservoirs have the remains of old forests in them. They will look like dead trees sticking straight up out of the water. When fishing these areas, try to find the flooded tree that is a little bit different from its neighbors. For some reason, fish seem to prefer trees that stand out a bit. It could be because it's an easy way for the fish to spot their home, or maybe they just have their own sense of style!

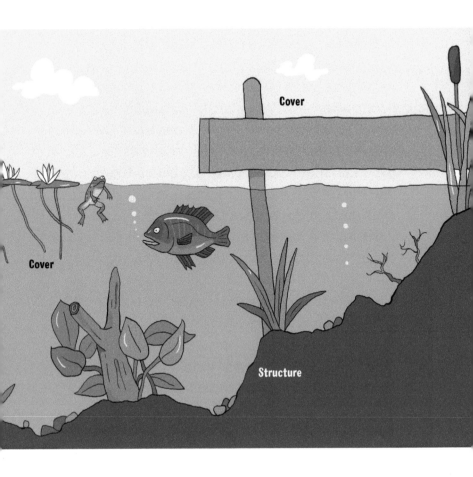

Cover

Cover

Structure

STRUCTURE

Bays: These are flat protected areas along the edges of a body of water. They usually have a muddy or sandy bottom and often are full of weeds like lily pads and bullrushes. They tend to hold fish all year round, but are best for fishing in the spring and summer. Many types of fish spawn in bays to raise their young in the protected waters. Plastic worms and spinnerbaits work very well in these areas.

Points: A point is a piece of land that juts into the water. A jetty would be an example of a man-made point, but they can also occur naturally. Points with lots of rocks can be some of the best places to fish early in the year, especially if they are near a bay. Some fish, like largemouth bass, like to gather on these rocky points just before they move into the bays to spawn. Crankbaits and jerkbaits work great on rocky points.

Humps: A hump is an underwater hill. Fish like to gather on these, especially if they have cover. If a hump breaks the surface, it is called an island. In reservoirs that have very steep banks, humps are some of the best places to fish.

Channels: A channel is basically an underwater path or ditch that is deeper than the surrounding areas. This deeper water is cooler and allows fish to hide. Channels can be great places to find big fish, especially if they're near the mouth of a creek.

Fishing from a Boat

Have you ever tried fishing from a boat? It completely changes the sport. While I do enjoy fishing from shore, I love the many options a boat provides. A boat lets you put yourself exactly where you need to be to cast exactly where you want.

A fishing boat doesn't have to be fancy. As long as weather conditions are calm, any rowboat or canoe with an anchor can bring you to a good fishing spot and hold you there while you fish. Some people even prefer small watercraft like canoes and kayaks because they are much quieter, making it easy to sneak up on fish. While small boats are fun, they are tippy. It can be dangerous to stand on a tippy boat. If the boat wobbles when you try to stand up, fish sitting down instead.

If you are fishing from a boat, here are a couple of different ways to do it.

→ You can drive the boat to your favorite fishing spot and throw out the anchor. This works well in areas that hold many fish, or when you want to fish slowly with a worm or bobber. You can often put your boat in an ideal position to cast to the perfect spot. Then you can just leave your bait there, waiting for a bite.

→ You can also drift in a boat. Drifting is when you let the wind push your boat through an area while you take casts along the way. You can cover a large area this way and ideally find some hungry fish. Drifting is a very useful way to figure out where the good spots are if you're new to a lake.

You might not always be on a boat with just a parent. Sometimes you might go on a charter boat or other larger boat. One challenge about fishing from a boat with other people is that it can get crowded quickly. All those people are there to fish, too, so the likelihood that a lure will hit you by

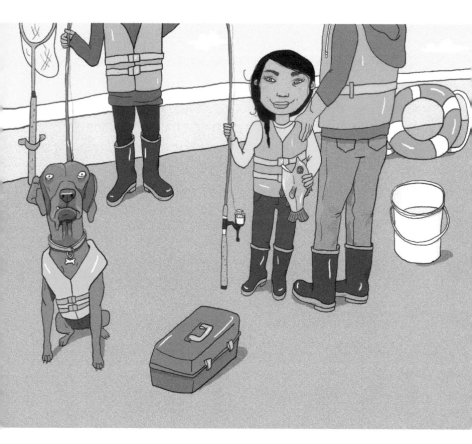

accident increases. Even if you aren't hit by a lure, there's a good chance that you and a fishing partner may cross lines and get tangled if you aren't careful. A good way to prevent these issues is to have everyone in the boat have a certain "zone" that they can cast to. For example, the person fishing in the front of the boat should cast toward the front while the person fishing in the rear should cast toward the back. This will take care of many problems.

If your boat is crowded, it's important to be aware of who is around you. What if you accidentally cast over someone else's line? Stop and assess the situation. Allow the person to reel in their line before you start reeling in yours. Otherwise, you'll end up snagging their line with your hook and cause a tangle.

Another thing to remember when fishing from a boat is that it's important to be neat and tidy. There is not much space, so it is important that you have your net in a place that is out of the way but can be reached if needed. Make sure you don't take more gear than you need and put it away after you use it. The last thing anyone wants to do is trip over a bag and get hurt or step on a rod and break it because of limited space.

> **SAFETY TIP** Most states have laws that require younger anglers (and older ones) to wear life jackets when they are on a boat. While states have somewhat different rules, I suggest that you always wear yours. The thing about life jackets is that they only work when you're wearing them, and you don't always know that you're about to need one. Even if you and the adult who is driving the boat are doing everything right, you could run into someone with less experience who makes a mistake and causes an accident. If you always wear your life jacket, you'll always be prepared.

PROTECTING FISH AND THEIR HOMES

It's important that we all do our part to protect the environments of fish and other animals. That means leaving fishing spots cleaner than we found them, handling fish with care, and only taking what we need from nature—never more.

Every now and then, you may hear a news story about an owl or other animal that got caught in fishing line. Please don't be the angler that leaves their line behind. If you get snagged on something, pull the line tight and give it a quick tug. It will usually snap near the snag rather than near your hand and you'll be able to save more of it. If you're using braid, remember to wrap the line around a big stick before you pull so you don't get hurt.

When you catch a fish, it's important to handle it with care. Most fish have a protective slime on their bodies that helps them stay healthy. Dry hands can rub off the slime easily, so wet your hands before you grab a fish. Larger fish should be supported by their bellies when you hold them. You can also consider the fish's health *before* you catch it by using barbless hooks that are less likely to injure it.

Finally, if you're planning to fish from a boat, be sure to bring proper sunscreen and gear. When you're on a boat there is usually no shade. The sun's glare also reflects off the water and onto your skin. If you don't wear sunscreen and other sun gear, your fun fishing trip could turn into a painful memory.

Fishing from a boat can be exciting and a great way to catch some **keepers**. But, as always, don't feel bad if you don't have a boat you can use. There are plenty of great fishing spots that you can reach right from shore.

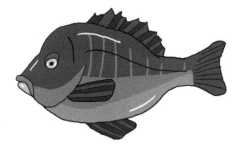

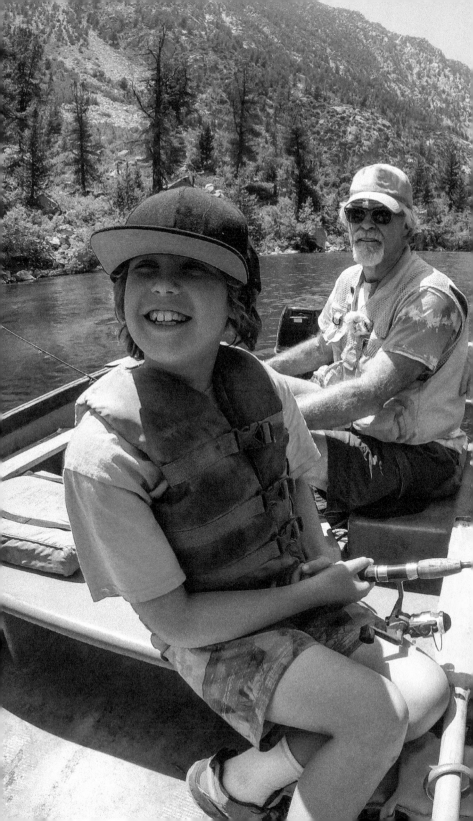

CHAPTER THREE

Let's Catch Fish!

This chapter is where "the rubber meets the road," or "where the lure hits the water." Things are about to get exciting! You are going to put the skills you learned in the first two chapters to work. We'll talk about how to bait a hook, set your drag, take a cast, set the hook, fight, and land a fish. We'll also spend a little time discussing the practices of **catch and release** as well as **selective harvest**, so you can figure out which fish to keep for a meal. Finally, you'll learn how to clean your fish and prepare it for the table.

59

SPRINKLED THROUGHOUT THIS

chapter you'll find several Fish Facts. These are snippets of information that will help you on your angling journey. These little tips can save you a lot of time and trouble, so make sure you read them.

How to Bait a Hook

You're not going to catch many fish with a bare hook, so you'd better learn how to properly bait one. There are different ways to do this. The basic idea is that you want to get your bait on tight, but also allow it to move around, which excites the fish and makes it want to bite.

If you're using a worm, spear the worm through the head and then thread the hook through its body. If you're going for bigger fish, you'll want to leave more of the worm's tail free to dangle in the water. Unfortunately, smaller fish will often bite off the tail before a bigger fish can come by. When fishing for smaller fish, it often makes sense to only use part of a worm. Thread it onto the hook right near the point.

▶️ BARBLESS HOOKS ON THE FLY

Barbless hooks are much safer for fish. You don't have any? No problem. You can make almost any hook barbless by pinching the barbs with a pair of pliers.

If you're using a minnow, bait the hook right through its mouth. This allows the fish to move its tail and swim around a bit, which will attract bites. Some people hook their minnows just under the dorsal fin, which is the fin on top of the body, because they believe this keeps them on the hook better.

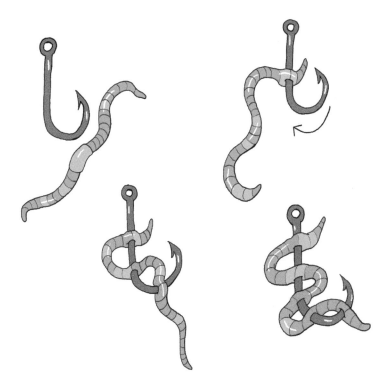

If fishing with live bait is not something you want to do, you could use soft plastics (see page 27). These often look just like the real thing and can be baited the same way. When using artificial worms, there are two main techniques for rigging them: the wacky rig (see page 25) and the Texas rig.

To use a Texas rig, push the hook through the tip of the worm's head but at an angle, so it almost immediately comes out. Push the hook through the worm up to the eye of the hook. Then, twist the hook around and bury its point into the middle of the worm. Because the hook is buried in the worm, your lure will glide through weeds with very little snagging.

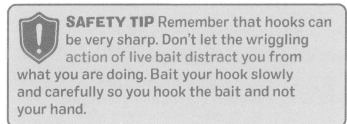

SAFETY TIP Remember that hooks can be very sharp. Don't let the wriggling action of live bait distract you from what you are doing. Bait your hook slowly and carefully so you hook the bait and not your hand.

Setting the Drag

Before you take your first cast, it's important to set the drag on your reel properly. What is the drag? It is a set of friction plates inside the reel that control how easy it is to pull out line. The drag has two important jobs:

→ It helps prevent your line from breaking.

→ It helps tire out fish you are fighting, and allows you to reel them in.

When your drag is properly set, a fish will have to work hard to take line from the reel. It won't be able to snap it because the drag will give way before the line reaches its breaking point.

Most spinning reels have a little knob or dial either on the top of the spool or toward the bottom of the reel. Turn this dial to the right to tighten the drag, and to the left to loosen it. The drag on most baitcasters is a plastic or metal star-shaped knob on the side of the reel. Again, turn this knob to tighten or loosen it.

To check how tight your drag is, take some line in your hand and give a little tug. Remember to be careful about doing this with braid, as it can cut

►●○ HOW MUCH TIME IS THERE LEFT TO FISH?

Hold your flat hand up between the horizon and the sun making sure your fingers are parallel to the horizon. Each finger between the horizon and sun represents 15 minutes of fishing time before dark.

you. You want the line to give a little and pull out, but you also want to feel some resistance. Setting your drag too tight will cause your line to snap, but if it's too loose it can allow a fish to escape, taking all your line with it.

How to Cast

Your hook is baited. The drag is set. It's finally time to cast. Your casting technique depends on what type of reel you are using. Let's discuss how to cast the three most common reels: spinning reels, spincast reels, and baitcasting reels.

HOW TO CAST A SPINNING REEL

Casting a spinning reel can be a little tricky at first, but you'll get the hang of it quickly.

1. Grasp the rod near the reel and use the index finger of that hand to apply pressure to the line coming out of the reel. This will keep the line in place when you open the bail in step 2.

2. Use your other hand to open the bail. Don't stop applying pressure to the line, as discussed in step 1.

3. Carefully pull the rod back and to the side.

4. In one smooth movement, cast the rod forward.

5. When your rod tip is pointed in the direction that you want the lure to go, release the line from your pointer finger. The lure will sail forward and eventually splash down.

6. Close the bail with your hand. You could reel in to close it, but this is bad for the reel and you will wear it out sooner.

HOW TO CAST A SPINCAST REEL

Spincast reels are easier to cast than spinning reels because you don't have to worry about holding any line with your index finger. Instead, they have a button that you press in and hold until you are ready to release the line at the end of a cast.

1. Grasp the rod near the reel while pressing down the button on the reel with your thumb. Do not release the button.

2. Pull the rod back and to the side, just as you would with a spinning rod.

3. In one smooth movement, cast the rod forward.

4. When the rod tip is pointed in the direction you want the lure to go, take your thumb off the button.

5. Once the lure splashes down, turn the handle to start reeling in.

HOW TO CAST A BAITCASTING REEL

Baitcasting reels are challenging to learn to cast. As I've said before, I don't recommend them for beginners, but you may want to try them one day since they are more precise and powerful.

1. Grasp the handle with your hand around the reel and place the tip of your thumb firmly on the spool to apply pressure on the line.

2. With the base of your thumb, press the spool release button. Do not lift the tip of your thumb off the reel.

3. As with other types of reels, make a cast by pulling the rod back, and then smoothly moving it forward.

4. When you want to release your lure, take your thumb off the spool for a moment. Now for the tricky part . . .

5. "Thumb" the spool by resting your thumb lightly on the line as the spool turns. This will slow down the spool so it doesn't rotate faster than the line is coming off of it.

6. Just as the lure splashes into the water, press your thumb firmly on the spool to stop it from turning.

If you don't succeed with steps 5 and 6, you may get the worst tangle you have seen in your entire life. Casting into the wind makes it extremely likely that this will happen.

OVERHAND VS. SIDEARM CASTS

I've talked about casting the line, but how exactly do you do that? Two common techniques are overhand and sidearm. If you've ever played hockey, an overhand cast is very much like a slap shot, while a sidearm cast uses the same muscles and techniques as a wrist shot.

An overhand cast is powerful and can make your lure fly far but isn't always accurate. It is also more difficult to use from shore because of the risk of snagging trees. To use an overhand cast, raise your rod straight up over your head and behind. Then move it forward quickly toward the water.

A sidearm cast is more accurate and useful than an overhand cast. To use a sidearm cast, move your rod back and to your side. Then flick your wrists to send the lure flying toward the water.

You should try practicing casting a plug in your backyard until you get the hang of things. If you do this, remember to take off the hooks first.

SAFETY TIP Before you take a cast, do everyone near you a favor and look around. You don't want to accidentally snag your fishing buddy. Make sure you have enough room before you pull your rod back. Even if you are fishing alone, you should still get in the habit of doing this so you don't accidentally hook a bush or tree.

WHEN THE FISH WON'T BITE

Every angler has a day now and then when the fish just won't bite. This can happen for many reasons, most of which are completely out of your control. Maybe there is a sudden change in weather. Perhaps a fishing tournament from the day before scared all the fish. There's nothing you can do about either of these situations. While we'd all like to pick the perfect days to go fishing, most of us can only go on weekends or other days off. Sometimes the conditions are not ideal on those days.

Rather than worrying about what you can't change, focus on what you can change. First, figure out if you're fishing too aggressively. When fishing conditions are tough, large lures are poor choices. Try something smaller and simpler, then take it slow.

You can also try moving to another fishing spot. If you're not catching any fish on rocky points, maybe they're in deep weeds in the bay. If they're not biting in shallow water, is it possible they went deep? Could a more dull-colored lure do the trick? How about a different lure entirely? Don't be afraid to mix things up until you find a pattern that works.

The best fishing spots often have multiple types of cover. You're usually better off fishing a bay that has many types of weeds instead of just one.

Setting the Hook

You've cast your line and feel a bite. What should you do next? Setting the hook is one of the most important steps for catching a fish. If you do it incorrectly, you risk losing the fish. "Setting the hook" means driving the hook into the fish's mouth to make a secure connection between the fish, hook, line, rod, and you. It is important that this connection is as strong as possible, so do your best.

The first step is to realize that you have a fish biting in time to do something about it. If you are using live bait, wait until you see either the bobber go underwater or the fishing line start to move, or you feel a tug.

Once you notice any of these, it's important to quickly reel in any loose line to make a tight connection. As soon as you can feel the connection with the fish, it can feel it with you and will try to do something about that. You need to act fast. What you do depends on the type of hook you are using.

If you are using a bait or lure with a large, thick hook (like a spinnerbait or plastic worm) you need to snap the rod back toward you HARD. Do this by quickly raising your rod toward the sky and back. It takes a lot of force to drive a large, thick hook into a fish's mouth.

If your bait or lure has very thin hooks (like treble hooks or light wire hooks you might use with a drop shot), you need to sweep your rod back in one smooth motion. It doesn't take as much force for one of these hooks to pierce the fish's mouth. In this case, you should be careful not to tear your hook completely out of its mouth.

If you are using a circle hook, then you don't set the hook at all. These hooks are designed to catch the very corner of the fish's mouth when you reel in your line. Attempting to set the hook by snapping your rod back can fail and you may pull the whole rig away from a fish.

Sometimes you may get lucky and fish will bite a lure so hard that it hooks itself, but you can't count on this. Do the best you can and realize that you aren't going to catch them all. You can always try to catch them again another day.

▶☰◦ POLARIZED GLASSES

Sunglasses aren't just for keeping the sun out of your eyes. If they're polarized, they cut down on sun glare, letting you see into the water better.

Playing the Fish

After you've set the hook, it's time to play the fish. "Playing the fish" means tiring it out enough while reeling it in so you can land, or capture, it. There is a balance here because you want to tire out the fish enough to safely grab it, but not injure it. Playing the fish is an art more than it is a science. This means what you do depends on the situation. There is not one way that will work all the time. That said, there are a few basic rules to follow. Here are three of them.

DON'T REEL IN WHILE THE FISH IS TAKING A RUN

It's not a good idea to reel in your line while a fish is taking a run, which means "swimming away." This puts a lot of pressure on the line and may cause it to snap. It can also cause your line to twist, which will create tangles later. When a fish is running, keep a bend in your rod and let it take line. If you set your drag correctly, as discussed on page 63, then the fish will tire itself doing this. If you're worried that the fish is heading for cover, which it probably is, try to

▶️ FLOAT PLAN

Always tell your parents or a friend where you plan to fish and when you'll be back. This way, if something happens, someone will come look for you.

►⬤ BURNING SPINNERBAITS

When you find submerged weeds below the water's surface, "burn" a spinnerbait on top of them by reeling fast. Northern pike won't be able to resist.

pull it away from the cover using the rod, if possible. Start reeling once it stops running or when your line becomes slack, or loose.

ALWAYS KEEP PRESSURE ON THE FISH

When I was a little kid, my dad would always tell me, "Keep your rod up high!" whenever I was playing a fish. This is not the best idea sometimes because it can encourage a fish to jump and can even break your rod. The reason he told me this was because he wanted me to keep pressure on the line. You want to *always* feel the fish's weight while you are playing it. The second you don't feel its weight, there is slack in the line. This slack can let the hook change position and fall out.

DON'T POINT YOUR ROD TIP DIRECTLY AT THE FISH

Your fishing rod is meant to bend. This bend absorbs some of the shock that a fighting fish puts on your line. If you point your rod directly at the fish, your rod can no longer absorb this shock. As a result, you are now relying entirely on the strength of your line, which may snap.

Landing the Fish

You are almost there! Once you have played the fish and reeled it to the shore or boat, it is time to land it. When you land a fish, you capture it and bring it out of the water. The first step when landing a fish is playing it to the point where it is tired enough be taken from the water. Just because a fish is right next to the boat or shore does not mean that it is ready to come in. If you try to force it, there is a good chance you'll lose the fish. Be very aware of this when trying to land larger fish like northern pike. They are famous for making last-minute runs near the boat. Make sure the fish has stopped making too many jerks or runs before you try to grab it.

Once the fish is ready to be landed, hold your rod with one hand while reaching for the fish with the other hand, with a net if possible. Make sure that you keep the line tight while you do this because otherwise the fish might wiggle off the hook.

Some people like to land fish with their hands. While there aren't many other options if you leave your net at home, this is a great way to get hurt and I don't recommend it. One sharp movement from a fish is all it takes for you to become hooked, too. If you do have to land a fish by hand, know what species you're dealing with. *Never* put your hand in the mouth of a fish you don't recognize, as some fish have very sharp teeth.

It's always safer for you and the fish to use a net, but not just any net will do. Nets that are made of untreated rope can injure fish. It's better to buy a net that has a protective rubber coating; it won't scrape off as much slime or injure the fish as badly as a rope one will.

When using a net, lead the fish into it headfirst. If you try to net a fish tailfirst, it will panic when its tail touches the net, and it will try to jump out. Don't poke at the fish with the net either, as you can knock it off the hook. Instead, scoop the fish up in one smooth motion.

Whatever you do, never drag a fish onto the shore. Remember that protective slime coat discussed in chapter 2? There's nothing like rocks and sand for scraping it off.

▶ SOLVING A SLIPPERY BAIT PROBLEM

Some bait, like chicken liver, is hard to keep on the hook. Solve this problem by making a little pouch out of some used nylon stocking.

CATCH AND RELEASE

If every angler who visited a pond kept every fish they caught, it wouldn't be long before there weren't any fish left. As you get better at fishing, it will become more and more important that you release many of the fish that you catch so they can be caught another day. In some cases it's the law, such as at lakes that have a limit on how many fish an angler may keep. Even if it isn't the law where you fish, it's a good idea to practice catch and release, or at least selective harvest.

It does little good to release fish that are too injured to survive, so it's important that you are careful when you catch them and take care of them once they're caught. Here are some simple and important rules to follow.

→ Use barbless hooks. They don't hurt the fish as badly and are much easier to remove.

→ To remove a hook, grip the fish firmly in one hand and use pliers with the other hand to remove the hook. This is safer, quicker, and better for all involved.

→ Use proper tackle that can land fish quickly. While it might be "more fun" to catch a big fish on light gear, it stresses the tackle out more and makes the fish more likely to get hurt. Land fish quickly.

→ When you do catch a fish, remember to wet your hands before you handle it so you don't wipe off its protective slime. Also, touch it as little as possible for this same reason.

→ Try your best to get the fish back in the water as quickly as possible.

→ Support the fish's weight while taking photos. If it is a large fish, consider holding its belly as well as its mouth.

→ When you release the fish, do so gently. Place it in the water; don't toss it in like a football.

▶● CALMING SMALLMOUTH BASS

Smallmouth bass are famous for fighting. It can be difficult to land them without a net, but if you cradle them by the belly they will calm down.

MY FISH SWALLOWED THE HOOK! NOW WHAT?

There will come a day when a fish swallows a hook so far down its throat that you won't think you can get it back. You have several options to try to deal with this. Some are better for the fish than others.

What you *don't* want to do—ever—is tug on the line to try to rip out the hook. If you do this, you will likely kill the fish.

You can either leave the hook in the fish or remove it. If you cannot see the hook or the fish is bleeding, I recommend cutting the line as close to the hook as possible and letting the fish go. Many hooks will wiggle their way out or rust out over time. At least this gives the fish a fighting chance.

If you want to try to remove it, turn the hook in such a way that the eye of the hook is facing the fish's tail while you pull the hook out by its bend. Do this by moving the eye of the hook toward or out of the **gill plates** and then pulling on the hook with pliers from its bend.

If you don't want to be in this situation, consider using circle hooks. They are designed specifically to prevent fish from swallowing them.

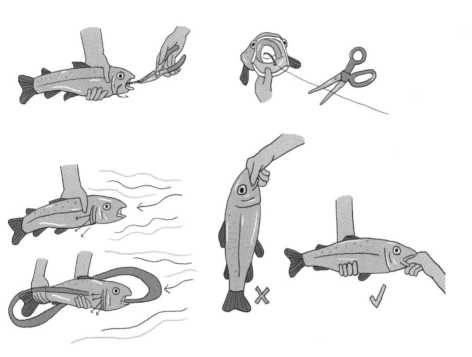

SELECTIVE HARVEST

Where it's legal, there is nothing wrong with keeping some of your catch to eat, but you should carefully select the fish you take home to protect the species. Consider the largemouth bass, for example. It is incredibly rare for a bass to live long enough to grow to be five pounds. Those that do grow that large should have the chance to have babies who may share the qualities that made their parents successful. Rather than keeping the one biggest fish you catch, it often makes sense to keep two or three medium-size ones. This is called selective harvest. It will help ensure good fishing for years to come. Smaller fish also tend to taste better, so it's a win-win!

CARING FOR YOUR CATCH

You've spent the day fishing and caught some fish. Now, you want to bring some home to cook for dinner. There's nothing wrong with keeping a portion of your catch to eat. Human beings are natural fish predators and have been catching and eating them for as long as we've been on Earth. Fish make a delicious and nutritious meal, and it can be both fun and rewarding to help your family by catching dinner.

Even so, there is no mistaking the hard truth of the matter: You must end a fish's life before eating it. You should do this as humanely as you can. A humane death is quick and as painless as possible so the fish doesn't suffer. This process starts right after you catch your fish.

If you plan on cleaning your fish on the boat, make sure you have ice to store the meat. If you plan on cleaning your fish when you get back to shore, you will need a place to keep them as calm as possible. The fish will need to be in water. If you are on a boat that has a tank with water, called a live well, that is best. Put the fish in, close the lid, and remember to keep changing the water throughout the day. Putting a live fish on ice to store it is not humane, so don't ever do this.

If you are fishing from shore, bring a bucket and fill it with water. Keep the bucket and the fish out of the sun. If you don't have a bucket, you'll need to make a stringer of some kind. A stringer can be as simple as a piece of rope that you put through the fish's mouth and then out its gill plate before tying the rope into a knot so the fish can't slide off. Tie the other end to a tree branch and keep

▶ REPLICA MOUNTS

Rather than killing a fish to stuff and mount it, consider having an environmentally friendly fiberglass replica made instead.

the fish in the water until you are ready to kill it and go home.

The most humane way to kill a fish is by stunning it first. Do this by hitting it firmly on the head with a hard, heavy object like a rock. This will knock the fish unconscious so it won't feel pain. After you are sure the fish is stunned, use a knife to cut through the fish's gills to kill it. The fish will bleed, so make sure that you do this someplace you don't mind getting messy.

Ending a life isn't easy and this can be a disturbing process. Don't feel pressured into doing it if you don't want to or aren't comfortable. There are plenty of fish in the supermarket. But if you do decide to keep your catch, please follow these guidelines for the sake of the fish.

HOW TO CLEAN A FISH

Before you can eat a fish, you need to clean it, which means preparing it for cooking or storage. Basically, you will remove the parts of the fish you can eat and discard the rest. Some boat ramps and fishing spots have a hut or table where you can clean your fish, but if not, you may need to do

►●▷ THE ONE-TWO PUNCH

If you're fishing with a spinnerbait or topwater lure and a fish attacks it and misses, try casting a plastic worm to that same spot. Often, you'll get a second chance at that fish.

Don't be afraid to work an area thoroughly. Sometimes it takes many casts before a fish will commit to an attack. Try casts from multiple angles until you find one that works.

this at home. I strongly discourage doing this on your family's antique dining table!

To clean a fish, you will need a sharp knife. There is a special type of knife called a fillet knife, and it is the best one for this job. If you don't have one, though, use a sharp knife with a long, thin blade. Be extremely careful with the knife when you are using it.

To clean the fish, follow these steps:

1. Rinse the fish with cold water.

2. Pat it dry with a clean paper towel and place it on a hard cutting surface.

3. Lift the pectoral fin, which is the first fin on either side of the fish behind its head.

4. Place your knife right behind the pectoral fin, and angle it toward the fish's head.

5. Cut down and toward the head until you feel the backbone.

6. Turn your knife toward the tail of the fish and cut along the backbone to the tail. A sawing motion helps.

CUTTING INTO FISH

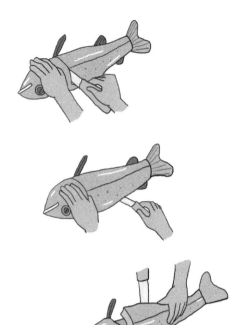

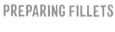
PREPARING FILLETS

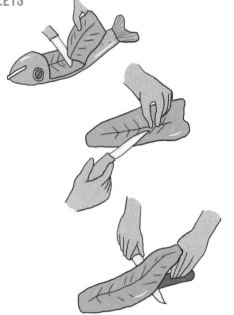

Repeat this process with the other side of the fish. When you are done, you will have two fillets, but they might not be ready to eat. Different fish species can have a lot of fat that needs to be trimmed or a row of bones that you'll want to try to cut out. Take your time so you don't lose more meat than necessary.

If you can't fillet a dead fish within a few hours, you'll need to field dress it. This is simply removing the gills, guts, and kidneys, since these will spoil fast in dead fish and make the meat taste bad. To field dress a fish, cut out the red gills, then make a slice down its belly from back to front. With the belly open, remove the intestines and any organs that you see. This will buy you some time before you can fillet the fish properly.

> **SAFETY TIP** Fish are slippery, and knives are sharp. This can be a bad combination. Always make sure that an adult is present with a first aid kit to supervise and assist you while you are cleaning a fish.

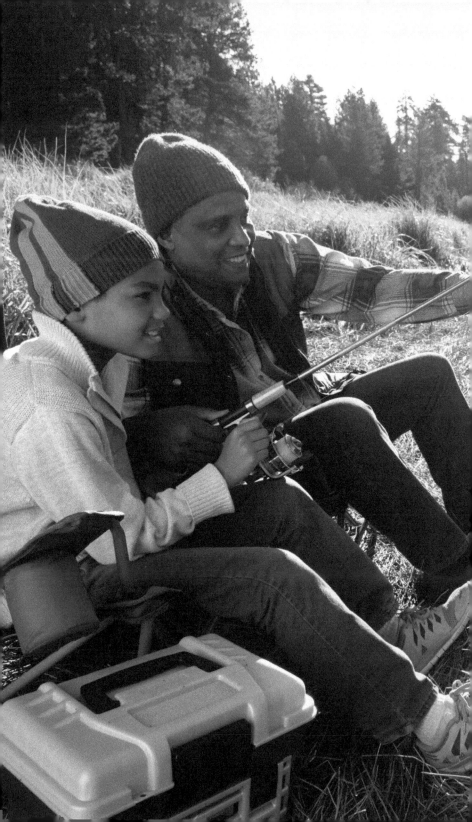

CHAPTER FOUR

Meet the Freshwater Fish

So, what kinds of fish can you expect to catch on your freshwater fishing adventures? You are about to find out. In this chapter I'll dive into some of the most common freshwater species you're likely to catch and give you some tips for how to catch them. There are too many fish to list here, but you can check out the Resources section for books and websites that discuss more fish and ways to catch them.

YOU'LL NOTICE THAT THERE IS A
fishing log at the end of this chapter. Use it
to record your catches so that you'll have
information you can use in the future. One of
the toughest parts of any fishing trip is
figuring out what to do. If you keep detailed
notes in this log, you can always look back
and see what worked before. Now it's time to
meet some fish.

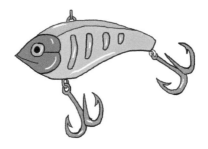

Largemouth Bass

Largemouth bass are one of anglers' favorite fish to catch. These fish fight hard, jump, dive, and are just really fun on the line. Largemouth bass hang out in weed beds and shallow bays but can go much deeper in some southern reservoirs. True to their name, these fish have such big mouths that some people call them "bucketmouths." These bass are usually shades of light to dark green and have a dark stripe along each side of their bodies. They will strike any lure described in this book, but it's hard to beat a simple plastic worm.

REGIONS: Common in most of the United States

SIZE: Up to 20 pounds; more commonly 1 to 5 pounds

HABITAT: Weedy bays, slow-moving water

FOOD: Fish, frogs, crayfish

TACKLE: Medium to medium-heavy power rods

BAIT: Plastic worms, jigs, spinnerbaits, crankbaits

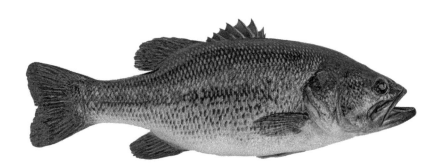

Smallmouth Bass

Many anglers think that, for their size, smallmouth bass are the hardest-fighting fish in North America. This largemouth's smaller cousin is usually found in clear water or fast-moving streams. They're known for schooling and traveling great distances. Smallmouth bass are a bronze or brown color, which is why some people call them "bronzebacks" or "footballs." All the lures that catch largemouth will also catch these fish, though you may want to downsize a bit.

REGIONS: Common in most of the United States

SIZE: Up to 11 pounds; more commonly 1 to 4 pounds

HABITAT: Rocky cover and riprap

FOOD: Smaller fish, crayfish, insects

TACKLE: Medium tackle with at least 6 lb. line

BAIT: Drop shot minnows, crankbaits, jerkbaits

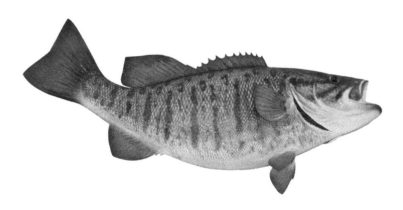

Sunfish

Bluegills, pumpkinseeds, and other sunfish are probably the first fish you ever caught. These small fish have huge appetites and aren't afraid to peck away at bait on a hook. Their fierce nature and large numbers make them great fish to target, plus they're easy to catch. You can find them in shallow bays near weeds throughout the year. In spring, they like to hang out near bass nests.

COMMON SPECIES: Bluegill, pumpkinseed, redear sunfish, longear sunfish, rock bass

REGIONS: Across North America

SIZE: Up to about 12 inches; more commonly 4 to 8 inches; weight varies

HABITAT: Shallow areas with vegetation or other cover

FOOD: Insects, small fish

TACKLE: Light or even ultralight tackle

BAIT: Night crawlers or small jigs (marabou jigs, grubs, etc.)

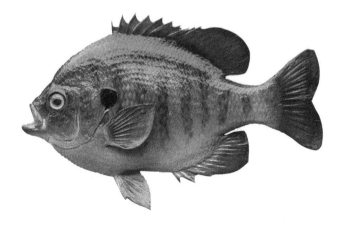

Yellow Perch

Yellow perch are a favorite of ice anglers as well as anyone who wants a delicious lunch. They are shaped like little walleye but are yellow with dark green vertical stripes on their bodies. They can be quite aggressive and are easy to catch using a small jig tipped with a worm. Perch are usually a schooling fish, so if you catch one, you'll likely catch more. Yellow perch are often in deeper water, which can make them tough to catch from shore depending on your area.

REGIONS: Northern United States and into Canada

SIZE: 4 to 10 inches; up to 4 pounds

HABITAT: Shallow weedy areas or slow-moving parts of rivers

FOOD: Insects, crayfish, small fish

TACKLE: Light or even ultralight tackle

BAIT: Night crawlers or small jigs (marabou jigs, grubs, etc.)

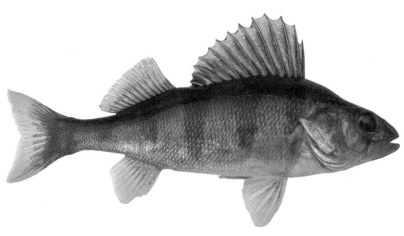

Crappie

Crappie or "calico bass" are a large, delicious panfish species that is fun to catch. Some people like fishing for them so much that there are rods, reels, and even boats designed just for them. Crappie can put up a great fight on light tackle and can grow large enough to grab bass lures. They're easy to tell apart from smaller sunfish because they tend to be silver with black spots or patches and have large mouths. Crappies love wooded cover, especially early in the spring.

REGIONS: Midwest to eastern United States

SIZE: Up to 3 or 4 pounds; more commonly 1 to 2 pounds

HABITAT: Clear, slow-moving water with weeds or wood for cover

FOOD: Crayfish, small fish, insects

TACKLE: Light tackle

BAIT: Night crawlers, small jigs, crankbaits

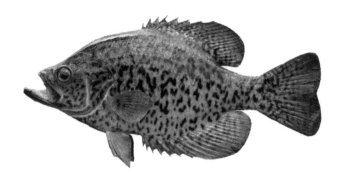

Catfish

Catfish tend to be some of the biggest fish in any given body of water. Have you ever hooked something so BIG that it eventually broke your line? Chances are it was a catfish. There are many species of catfish with slightly different colors and sizes, but they all have one thing in common—they have long whiskers like a cat's. Catfish will strike at lures, but a more common way to catch them is by using stink bait. Be careful when handling a catfish. The spines can poke you.

COMMON SPECIES: Channel catfish, blue catfish, flathead catfish, brown bullhead

REGIONS: Great Plains to the East Coast

SIZE: 3 to 6 pounds on average; 20 pounds or more are not uncommon

HABITAT: Slow-moving rivers and lakes

FOOD: Fish, mollusks, insects, crayfish

TACKLE: Heavy tackle

BAIT: Stink bait, chicken livers, night crawlers

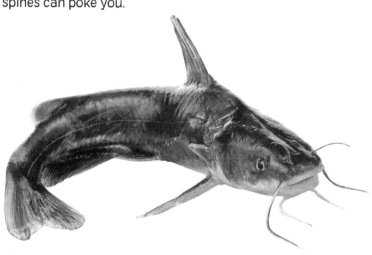

Trout

There are many species of fish called "trout" throughout the United States. Depending on where you are, they might be the main species you target. Some species, such as brook trout, are small. Others, such as rainbow trout, can grow to 50 pounds or more. Many species can be found in fast-moving rivers and are usually targeted by anglers using fly rods and reels. Local fish and game officers often stock lakes and rivers with trout because they are very popular targets.

COMMON SPECIES: Rainbow trout, brown trout, brook trout

REGIONS: Common throughout the United States

SIZE: 2 to 10 pounds are common; may be much larger

HABITAT: Cool water streams, some lakes

FOOD: Aquatic insects, leeches, small fish

TACKLE: Fly rods and gear or light spinning rods with light lures

BAIT: Flies, light inline spinners

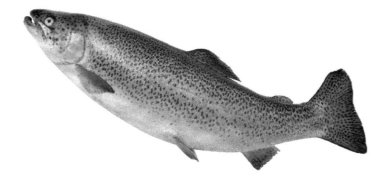

Walleye

This tasty fish is found throughout much of the Northeast and Midwest United States. In some states, it is a more popular target than largemouth bass. Walleye are members of the perch family and have the same basic shape, but walleye tend to be silver or light tan. These fish also have very distinct, bulging eyes that are made for hunting in low light conditions. Because of this, it's best to fish for walleye on cloudy days when the water is a little choppy.

REGIONS: Northern and central United States

SIZE: Up to 20 pounds; more commonly 4 to 8 pounds

HABITAT: Lakes and rivers; deep water during the day and shallow water in low light conditions

FOOD: Smaller fish, crayfish, leeches

TACKLE: Medium-light to medium tackle depending on lure

BAIT: Jigs tipped with leeches, deep-diving jerkbaits and minnows, grubs

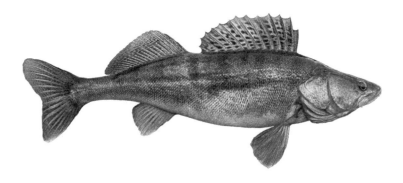

Northern Pike

If your fishing trip were a video game, a northern pike would be the final boss. As an **apex predator** in most places, northern pike eat whatever prey they want and can grow to be 20 pounds or more. During the summer, pike stay in deeper, cooler water but will move closer to shore in the spring and fall. Northern pike are long and slender and tend to be green with a series of white spots running along their sides. My kids call these "boo-boo fish" because of their razor-sharp teeth. Make sure you have an adult help you unhook one.

REGIONS: Northern and central United States

SIZE: Up to 20 pounds or more; more commonly less than 10 pounds

HABITAT: Natural lakes and rivers with access to cool water

FOOD: Fish, frogs, ducklings, small mammals

TACKLE: Medium-heavy or higher with strong line (20 lb. plus) and a wire leader

BAIT: Flashy, fast-moving lures

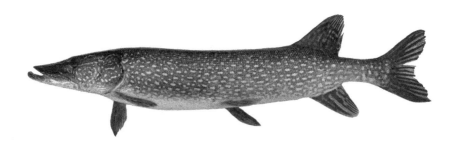

Chain Pickerel

Smaller cousins of the northern pike, chain pickerel are vicious feeders who will often strike fast-moving lures. Though the two species look similar, northern pike have many small, bean-shaped white spots and chain pickerel have a larger chain-like pattern on their bodies. These fish can usually be found in back bays or warmer waters throughout the summer. Chain pickerel can be extremely acrobatic once they're in the boat or net, so be careful when you go to unhook them. They often thrash around wildly once caught.

REGIONS: Southeast to eastern United States

SIZE: Up to 9 pounds; more commonly 2 to 4 pounds

HABITAT: Shallow bays in lakes and rivers; also in swamps and creeks

FOOD: Fish, frogs

TACKLE: Medium rods, at least 6 lb. line; a wire leader is helpful

BAIT: Spinnerbaits; plastic worms will work, but the fish may cut the line

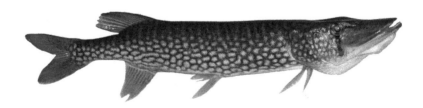

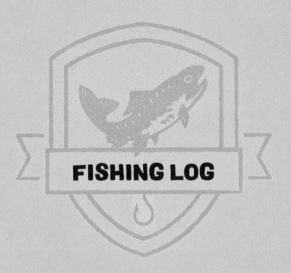

FISHING LOG

DATE: .... TIME: ....

LOCATION: ....

WEATHER: ....

FISHING WITH: ....

WHAT WORKED: ....

WHAT FAILED: ....

CATCH: ....

FISH	LENGTH	WEIGHT	LURE / BAIT

NOTES ....

....

....

SKETCH

DATE: .... TIME: ....

LOCATION: ....

WEATHER: ....

FISHING WITH: ....

WHAT WORKED: ....

WHAT FAILED: ....

CATCH: ....

FISH	LENGTH	WEIGHT	LURE / BAIT

NOTES ....

....

....

SKETCH

DATE: .... TIME: ....

LOCATION: ....

WEATHER: ....

FISHING WITH: ....

WHAT WORKED: ....

WHAT FAILED: ....

CATCH: ....

FISH	LENGTH	WEIGHT	LURE / BAIT

NOTES ....

....

....

SKETCH

DATE: .... TIME: ....

LOCATION: ....

WEATHER: ....

FISHING WITH: ....

WHAT WORKED: ....

WHAT FAILED: ....

CATCH: ....

FISH	LENGTH	WEIGHT	LURE / BAIT

NOTES ....

....

....

SKETCH

DATE: .... TIME: ....

LOCATION: ....

WEATHER: ....

FISHING WITH: ....

WHAT WORKED: ....

WHAT FAILED: ....

CATCH: ....

FISH	LENGTH	WEIGHT	LURE / BAIT

NOTES ....

....

....

SKETCH

DATE: .... TIME: ....

LOCATION: ....

WEATHER: ....

FISHING WITH: ....

WHAT WORKED: ....

WHAT FAILED: ....

CATCH: ....

FISH	LENGTH	WEIGHT	LURE / BAIT

NOTES ....

....

....

SKETCH

DATE: .... TIME: ....

LOCATION: ....

WEATHER: ....

FISHING WITH: ....

WHAT WORKED: ....

WHAT FAILED: ....

CATCH: ....

FISH	LENGTH	WEIGHT	LURE / BAIT

NOTES ....

....

....

SKETCH

DATE: .... TIME: ....

LOCATION: ....

WEATHER: ....

FISHING WITH: ....

WHAT WORKED: ....

WHAT FAILED: ....

CATCH: ....

FISH	LENGTH	WEIGHT	LURE / BAIT

NOTES ....

....

....

SKETCH

DATE: .... TIME: ....

LOCATION: ....

WEATHER: ....

FISHING WITH: ....

WHAT WORKED: ....

WHAT FAILED: ....

CATCH: ....

FISH	LENGTH	WEIGHT	LURE / BAIT

NOTES ....

....

....

SKETCH

DATE: .... TIME: ....

LOCATION: ....

WEATHER: ....

FISHING WITH: ....

WHAT WORKED: ....

WHAT FAILED: ....

CATCH: ....

FISH	LENGTH	WEIGHT	LURE / BAIT

NOTES ....

....

....

SKETCH

DATE: .... TIME: ....

LOCATION: ....

WEATHER: ....

FISHING WITH: ....

WHAT WORKED: ....

WHAT FAILED: ....

CATCH: ....

FISH	LENGTH	WEIGHT	LURE / BAIT

NOTES ....

....

....

SKETCH

DATE: .... TIME: ....

LOCATION: ....

WEATHER: ....

FISHING WITH: ....

WHAT WORKED: ....

WHAT FAILED: ....

CATCH: ....

FISH	LENGTH	WEIGHT	LURE / BAIT

NOTES ....

....

....

SKETCH

DATE: .... TIME: ....

LOCATION: ....

WEATHER: ....

FISHING WITH: ....

WHAT WORKED: ....

WHAT FAILED: ....

CATCH: ....

FISH	LENGTH	WEIGHT	LURE / BAIT

NOTES ....

....

....

SKETCH

DATE: .... TIME: ....

LOCATION: ....

WEATHER: ....

FISHING WITH: ....

WHAT WORKED: ....

WHAT FAILED: ....

CATCH: ....

FISH	LENGTH	WEIGHT	LURE / BAIT

NOTES ....

....

....

SKETCH

DATE: .... TIME: ....

LOCATION: ....

WEATHER: ....

FISHING WITH: ....

WHAT WORKED: ....

WHAT FAILED: ....

CATCH: ....

FISH	LENGTH	WEIGHT	LURE / BAIT

NOTES ....

....

....

SKETCH

DATE: .... TIME: ....

LOCATION: ....

WEATHER: ....

FISHING WITH: ....

WHAT WORKED: ....

WHAT FAILED: ....

CATCH: ....

FISH	LENGTH	WEIGHT	LURE / BAIT

NOTES ....

....

....

SKETCH

DATE: .... TIME: ....

LOCATION: ....

WEATHER: ....

FISHING WITH: ....

WHAT WORKED: ....

WHAT FAILED: ....

CATCH: ....

FISH	LENGTH	WEIGHT	LURE / BAIT

NOTES ....

....

....

SKETCH

DATE: .... TIME: ....

LOCATION: ....

WEATHER: ....

FISHING WITH: ....

WHAT WORKED: ....

WHAT FAILED: ....

CATCH: ....

FISH	LENGTH	WEIGHT	LURE / BAIT

NOTES ....

....

....

SKETCH

Good Luck, Anglers!

Well, anglers, that wraps up this book. I hope you've found it helpful and will keep it in your tackle box as a reference. I'm excited that you've decided to take up fishing and will become part of the next generation of conservationists protecting our great outdoors. That's an important responsibility, and I know you'll be up for the challenge.

Fishing isn't always easy. You won't catch something every time you go out, and you won't land every fish you hook. Even so, never give up! Make use of the log in this book, trust the knowledge that you've gained, and believe in yourself. You will catch far more than most.

Resources

This book is just one of many resources out there that can help you learn to fish. Here are some of my favorites.

Apps

Fishbrain.com This handy app lets you track your catches and see those of others. This is great for learning about new fishing spots quickly.

Fishidy.com Another app for local anglers to log their catches so others can learn where to have a better trip.

Websites

FHNBInc.org This is Fishing Has No Boundaries' official website. It offers tips and help for making fishing more accessible.

FishingFather.com My own website that is dedicated to teaching families how to fish.

Fishing.ScoutLife.org This website is geared toward kids who want to learn to fish and improve their fishing hobby.

In-Fisherman.com Visit this site to learn more about fishing specific species, gear, and even recipes for your catch. It covers all freshwater species in North America.

TakeMeFishing.org This great website focuses on learning how to fish, including fly fishing and even ice fishing.

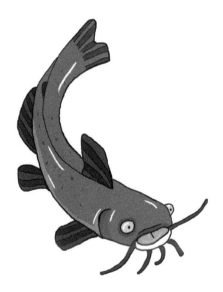

Glossary

angler: Someone who fishes with a fishing rod

apex predator: The top animal in the food chain with no natural predators

bail: The bar on a reel that keeps the line from unwinding from the spool and, when reeling in, guides it back onto the spool

catch and release: The act of letting a fish go immediately after catching it

chum: Little bits of food dumped into the water to attract fish to the area

cover: Objects such as rocks, weeds, or tree limbs that fish can hide in

drag: The system inside a reel that controls how easy it is to pull out line

eye: A circular ring on a rod that fishing line is fed through; also the hole in the top of fishing hooks

finesse fishing: A fishing technique that uses light lines and lures with only small movements

gill plate: The hard flap that covers and protects a fish's gills

keeper: A fish that is a legal size to keep

panfish: Any small edible fish that doesn't grow larger than a cooking pan

plug: A small wood or plastic lure shaped like a cylinder with treble hooks

rig: The equipment at the end of your fishing line that you are using to catch fish

selective harvest: The act of keeping several medium fish instead of the smallest or biggest fish

spawn: A time of year when fish mate and produce offspring

standing line: The fishing line that is coming off the reel's spool

strike: When a fish bites the lure or bait

structure: The ditches, valleys, and bumps that form the landscape underwater

tackle: All the rods, reels, lures, hooks, and gadgets anglers use to catch fish

tag end: The very end of the fishing line you are trying to tie

topwater lure: A lure that doesn't sink and stays on the water's surface

treble hook: A hook with three sharp points instead of one

trotline: A long fishing line tied across a river with multiple lines tipped with heavy hooks dangling from them

Index

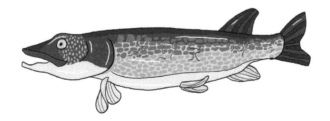

About the Author

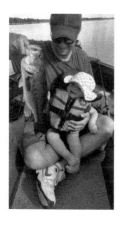

JOHN PAXTON is an avid angler who spends much of his time fishing with his two children across New England. John enjoys learning everything he can about fishing and boating, and shares what he learns on his website **FishingFather.com**. When he's not fishing or writing, he enjoys spending time with his wife, Crystal, and his two children, Tristan and Amber. In addition to this book, he is also the author of *Fishing with Kids: A Parent's Guide*. John can be reached at **johnpaxton@FishingFather.com**.

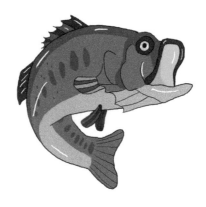

CPSIA information can be obtained
at www.ICGtesting.com
Printed in the USA
BVHW052346130921
616219BV00005B/3